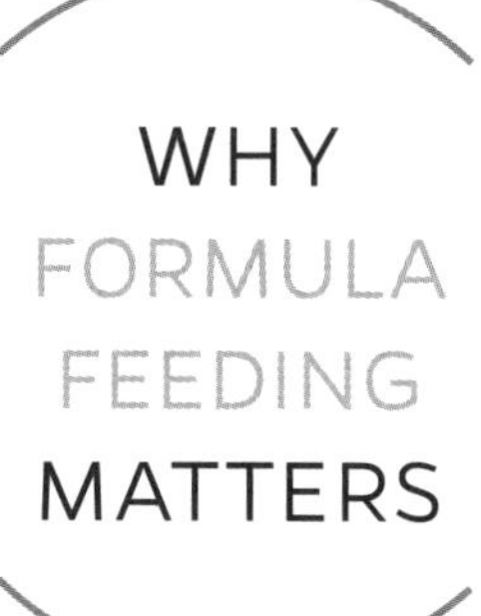
WHY
FORMULA
FEEDING
MATTERS

T0151138

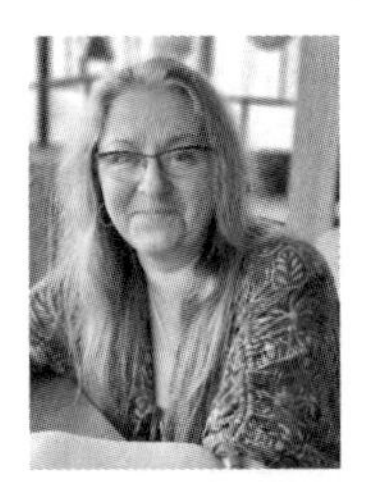

About the author

Shel Banks is an IBCLC and NHS infant feeding specialist based in Lancashire. She is vice-chair of the UK Association for Milk Banking, a charity which supports milk banks in the provision of donor human milk, and chair of LIFIB, which has been providing evidence-based information about formula and bottle-feeding to health professionals since 2008.

She is committed to evidence-based practice and the fully informed choice of expectant and new parents, and has contributed to three NICE Guidelines (Donor Milk Banking, Postnatal Care and Faltering Growth) and co-authored three Cochrane systematic reviews on various aspects of infantile colic.

Shel has a small private practice specialising in unsettled babies, disturbed sleep, formula feeding and faltering growth, and is a tutor for health and social care professionals in the UK and across the world.

Alongside teaching and coaching families and health professionals, Shel has also made a number of TV and radio appearances, including BBC Breakfast and the Channel 4 Dispatches documentary *The Great Formula Milk Scandal.*

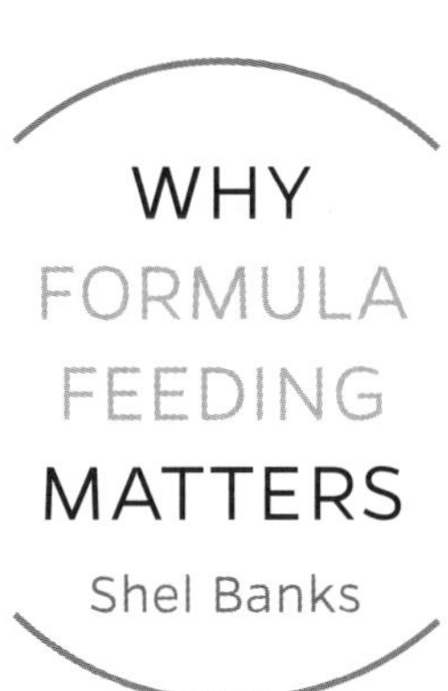
WHY
FORMULA
FEEDING
MATTERS
Shel Banks

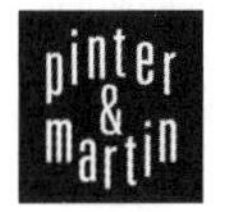
pinter
&
martin

Why Formula Feeding Matters (Pinter & Martin Why It Matters 23)

First published by Pinter & Martin Ltd 2022

ISBN 978-1-78066-595-5

Also available as an ebook

Pinter & Martin Why It Matters ISSN 2056-8657

Series editor: Susan Last
Index: Helen Bilton
Cover Design: Blok Graphic, London
Cover Illustration: Lucy Davey
Illustrations: Salma Price-Nell at thesalsacreative.com

British Library Cataloguing-in-Publication Data
A catalogue record for this book is available from the British Library.

Set in Minion

Printed and bound in the EU by Hussar

This book has been printed on paper that is sourced and harvested from sustainable forests and is FSC accredited.

Pinter & Martin Ltd
6 Effra Parade
London SW2 1PS

pinterandmartin.com

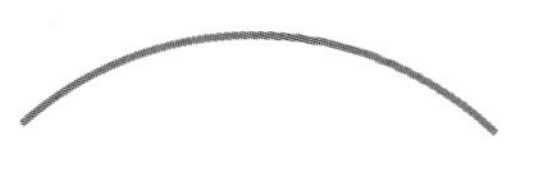

Contents

Author's note

This book is intended to help you make informed decisions about formula feeding. Whether you are already formula feeding or you are thinking about doing so, wholly or mixed with breastfeeding, what's important for your baby is that you have all the evidence-based information you need to do so as safely as possible.

I use the term 'parents' throughout this book, but I acknowledge that some readers may be carers of young bottle-fed infants, or supporters of families with new babies. The terms 'formula feed', 'infant milk' and 'bottles' are used fairly interchangeably; I know that the terms 'artificial feeding' and 'breastmilk substitute' can be uncomfortable to read, and so I have refrained from using these expressions except where required by the context.

Names and identifying details of individuals quoted in the book may have been anonymised at their request.

I am a fully qualified lactation consultant, not a medical doctor. The information in this book is not intended to take the place of expert and evidence-based information from your own medical professionals. If you have concerns about your own health or the health of your children, please consult a medical professional.

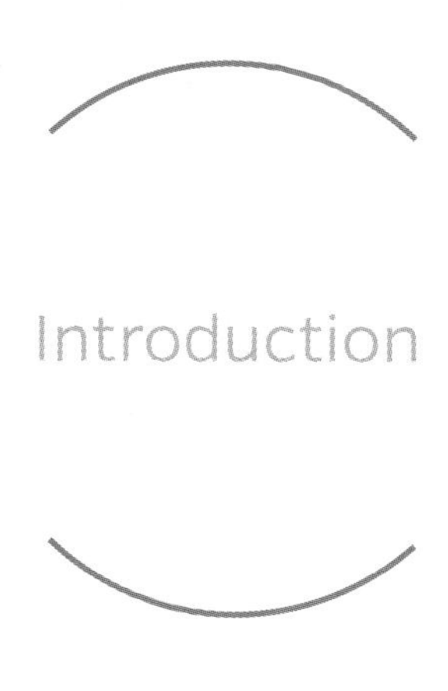

Introduction

First it seems fair to share a little bit about me. I have been supporting new parents with infant feeding online and in real life since 2001, and I trained as a breastfeeding peer supporter in 2002 and then qualified as an IBCLC (International Board Certified Lactation Consultant) in 2010. I am proud to be a Trustee of the UK Association for Milk Banking, I have worked in the NHS for 12 years and I have had a small private practice supporting families one-to-one since 2014.

You might be asking yourself why a lactation specialist is writing a book about formula feeding: why don't I stick to supporting breastfeeding?

Well, the short answer is that my overriding interest in providing unbiased and empowering information to families so that they can make their own decisions is not limited to those families who are breastfeeding. I want to support families to make well-informed decisions whatever their feeding journey looks like.

Actually, everyone who supports families with their new babies – including GPs, health visitors, peer supporters, doulas and so on – should be able to offer advice and support with formula feeding. They aren't just there for breastfeeding, so never be afraid to approach them with any questions you may have, and if the first person you contact can't help you, you can try someone else until you find the support you need.

Some more about me: I am passionate about the evidence base for our infant feeding decisions. I sat on the development committees of three NICE Guidelines, and have co-authored three Cochrane systematic reviews. I chair an organisation which looks at the evidence base for infant feeding-related things apart from breastfeeding, and I appeared on Channel 4's *Dispatches* programme in the UK talking about infant formula.

It frustrates me that many parents get their information about formula feeding from the formula companies' websites and helplines – these are definitely not unbiased, however 'balanced' they may seem at first glance – so I wanted to provide an alternative source of information that parents could access easily.

From my work with many, many families, I know that there is a strong feeling that there's not enough proper information and support for families who are partially or fully formula feeding, whether by choice or by circumstance, and I would like to do something to address that. My knowledge around perinatal mental health and health inequalities means that I would like all those working with families to know a lot more about formula feeding and how to effectively inform and support parents to care for their babies.

> *'I'd like to see proper info from the NHS online and face-to-face "feeding groups" – not just everything aimed at breastfeeding mums. All of what I've learnt has been from my own research.'* Heather

So, if you are reading this before your baby is born, and you would like some evidence-based information and sensible discussion about infant formula to help you make informed decisions about feeding your baby, this book is for you.

If your baby has already been born, and whether you had decided to formula feed from the get-go or whether you have found yourself formula feeding later on, this book is for you.

And if you are a health professional or someone working with expectant and new families, then there's plenty of information here to support you to support them, so this book is for you too.

> *'In comparison to my breastfeeding days with my first, formula feeding feels pretty lonely. Yes it's "easier" in many ways but it's also a minefield – what bottle, teat, formula to choose, how often and how much, how to troubleshoot issues.'* Heather

Let's have a look at some of the reasons you might be using infant formula.

Perhaps you have been advised to supplement or 'top up' a breastfed baby, due to weight-gain issues or other short term issues with breastfeeding – so you might need good information on how to protect your breastmilk supply (there are some signposts later in the book on where to go for great breastfeeding support if this is something you would like to continue) but you may well need a lot of the information in this book when making decisions about which formula to choose and how to feed it to your baby.

Perhaps you are having issues with breastfeeding and want to move towards mixed/combi feeding in the medium or long term. You might want to know how to balance this to ensure that you can continue breastfeeding alongside formula for as long as you want to, but you might also need information about formula. I often hear from families that they aren't really aware of mixed feeding as an option. Of course, you may feel that breastfeeding is simply not working for you and you want to stop, in which case you may benefit from information about how to how to do so safely and what and how to feed your baby instead.

> *'My husband had to rush out leaving me with a screaming baby to get some formula with no idea what to buy, and the midwife couldn't advise. I did have bottles and a steriliser which came with my pump – and which weren't prepped. I remember asking the midwife how to use a steriliser and she couldn't help me. It was very stressful combi feeding our baby but luckily he took to the bottle… I think it would have helped me to see formula as a supplement or 'medication' whereas I thought it was all or nothing. No one I saw then was equipped to help me with combi feeding.'* Claire

Perhaps you are returning to work or study and are planning to introduce formula partly or fully. You may have already been given information about how to protect your health by slowly reducing the amount of breastmilk you are producing, but now need information about how to gently transition to formula feeding, and to share with those who may be caring for your baby while you are away, about how and what to feed, and how to prepare, store and transport milk. It's also worth knowing that it's entirely possible to return to work or study without stopping breastfeeding, and there are signposts later in the book to sources of information and support on this, and on your rights as an employee.

Perhaps you are breastfeeding but feel that it would be

useful for baby to take an occasional bottle, and you want to have the flexibility for that bottle to be formula rather than expressed milk, but you don't know where to start with that. This book can provide you with information on how to make that work too.

Perhaps you have never entertained the idea of breastfeeding – you were always going to formula feed and it's what feels like the best fit for you, and of course that's fine. You may have tried to make informed decisions about which formula to use and found it tricky to get good information – the good news is that we have that covered in this book.

Ultimately, as an IBCLC I am keen for everyone to have all the information they need to confidently make decisions about feeding their infants. Of course I want parents to know how best to initiate and continue breastfeeding, and I became an IBCLC to offer support and information in that area, but the more time I spend working with families, the more I understand their experiences of the clear gap in information when it comes to those who are not fully breastfeeding, or who are not breastfeeding at all. I want to help bridge that gap.

Now let's look at some of the emotional considerations around formula feeding that I have come across while working with families over the last 20 years or so.

First of all, there's often a feeling of guilt, perhaps as a result of the pro-breastfeeding messages that abound. While breastfeeding is the biological norm for babies, many families feel that it isn't the right thing for them or for their specific circumstances. I often feel like guilt is such a waste of energy – if it cannot or will not change any action, then what's the point? As parents, we want to make the best decisions possible for our babies, and that needs to be done weighing up the pros and cons in that moment – no one likes to feel that they have made poor or ill-informed decisions, but as a mother with four teenagers I can tell you we are all winging it most of the time, doing the best we can in the circumstances.

If you were not intending to formula feed, then finding that you are no longer a breastfeeding parent can take you by surprise. The change in hormones when lactation ends or is ending can be very powerful and can make everything feel so much harder to deal with.

If people around you are not able to understand this wrench as your self-perception changes – perhaps they are trying to reassure you and to reduce your upset – you may hear such comments as 'all that matters is that she's healthy', or 'you're fine, he's fine – nothing to worry about', which are likely intended to make you feel better, but may actually make you feel worse. It's understandable for you to feel upset, to grieve, or to feel a little traumatised by the experience, and I want you to know you are not alone in this and it's okay to take some time to rebalance your feelings. There's an excellent book by Amy Brown, which is also part of the Pinter & Martin Why It Matters series, entitled *Why Breastfeeding Grief and Trauma Matter* – I have suggested it to many families and I know that it's been helpful. Debriefing with a trusted professional can also help enormously – you may not feel comfortable with an IBCLC or breastfeeding supporter, though we are all experienced in delivering this aspect of support – but a good postnatal doula might be just the person to talk it all through with, or a friend or family member who understands.

Of course, some parents were always intending to partially or totally formula feed and have zero issues with it – and that's great; if you are one such parent you might be wondering what all the fuss is about! I'd encourage you to read Amy Brown's book too – it's a real eye-opener and explains why the topic of feeding choice can be so divisive.

Overall, I want to make it clear that my stance is that

informed decisions help with feelings of confidence and can improve self-perception, so I work hard to make sure that parents have the information they need. Additionally, understanding and applying responsive feeding principles can really minimise any feelings of loss of relationship when breastfeeding is not happening, and is evidence-based best practice for all babies, which is why it's woven in throughout the book.

Finally, I wanted to end the beginning of this book with a look at what's coming up later on: we are going to talk about choosing formula, the differences between types, how to prepare it, the challenges of night-time parenting, troubleshooting issues and offering solutions, and many other issues. Let's get cracking!

A note about references

Throughout this book I refer to the evidence-based publications distributed by organisations including First Steps Nutrition Trust, the NHS and Unicef's Baby Friendly Initiative. These publications are fully referenced, so you can find the details of the scientific papers that form the evidence-base for formula feeding by consulting them. Information about how to interpret the research into formula feeding can be found in Chapter 9.

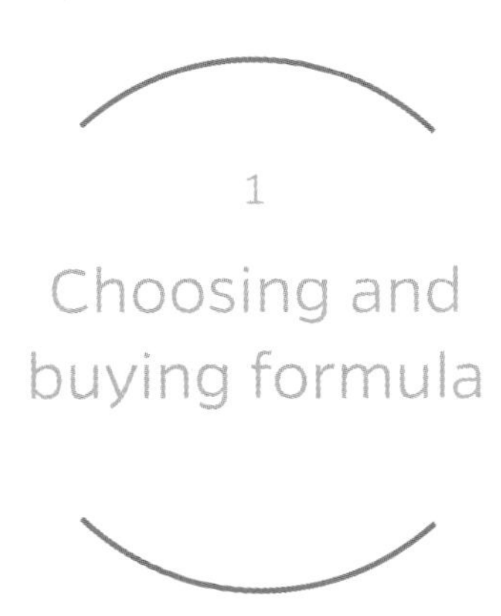

1 Choosing and buying formula

Choosing infant formula

The array of infant feeding products on the supermarket shelves can be overwhelming. Many parents wonder what all the products are *for* and some are interested to know what research and evidence supports them. Often families get in touch with me, or with their midwife, health visitor or GP, to ask which milk might be best for a particular baby or circumstance. Unfortunately there is no easy answer to this question. The ingredients of formula milks (apart from the ones controlled by legislation), and the claims for health benefits of different brands and formulations, change frequently. The best we can do is to say that since all formula must by law contain certain ingredients, you can choose based on price, availability, and what your baby seems to prefer. This can seem as though we are saying: '*it's your baby, your decision, and you are on your own!*' when the reality is that we all deserve better information about formula.

When there seems to be so much evidence-based

information available about breastfeeding, and breastfeeding mothers can access local peer supporters or even specialists to get breastfeeding working, parents can feel very lonely and unsupported when making choices about infant formula and bottles. It's no wonder so many new parents seek advice from their family and friends, or from online parenting groups.

Reading the packaging leaves us not much the wiser. Phrases such as 'unique blend of ingredients', 'inspiration taken from nature', 'delivering hard-to-get nutrients', 'contains nucleotides', 'can be used for combination feeding', 'makes bottle feeding easier', 'unique blend of oligosaccharides similar to those found in nature', 'LCPs and antioxidants', 'complete nutrition', 'the next generation of formula milk', 'certified organic', 'gentle', 'contains everything your baby needs for healthy development', 'tailored nutrient profile', and 'easy to digest' do not give us factual information that might be useful in decision-making.

Luckily there *are* some reliable and unbiased resources out there to help to demystify the products, their appropriate uses, and the evidence for their effectiveness. First Steps Nutrition Trust (www.firststepsnutrition.org) provides evidence-based information about all the main infant milks on the market in the UK, and updates the information whenever there's something new or the manufacturers make a substantial change to a product. Unfortunately this information is hard to come by, as the companies don't tend to let anyone know unless it's being used as a driver for marketing, and are often reluctant to provide the research studies which they claim have prompted the changes to their products. Where they do cite particular evidence it's possible to appraise the papers independently, which is ably done by First Steps Nutrition and to a lesser extent by bodies such as www.lifib.org.uk, which produces information, updates and training for health professionals, but has some consumer information too.

You might imagine that there would be a central requirement for the manufacturers of such important foodstuffs, essential to the survival and growth of so many of our nation's babies, to tell the public what is in their products, or to at least provide this information to a government department; but because it is classed as 'food', there is not. The standard infant milks have the same requirements for reporting contents on the packaging as any other processed or packaged food you can buy in the UK – a list of ingredients and a nutritional values table. Formula does have to conform to the maximum and minimum amounts of nutritional ingredients which are laid out in the European Food Standards Authority paper 'Scientific Opinion on the Essential Composition of Infant and Follow-on Formula' – more on that later in this chapter.

In the UK there are also rules about the guidance that must appear on the product's packaging about making up the milk. So standard infant milks in the UK carry guidance about using recently boiled water, because we know that the powder may be contaminated with bacteria and very hot water is needed to neutralise them. Alarmingly, the rules for specialist infant milks have less regulation – not more, as you might expect – because they are termed 'foods for special medical purposes'. They therefore do not carry the safer preparation information, although this is still very much applicable.

How is infant formula regulated?

The regulation that covers infant formula on sale in the UK is Regulation 2.16 of the Infant Formula and Follow-on Formula Regulations 2007, which you can find here: www.legislation.gov.uk/uksi/2007/3521/contents/made.

If you read it, you will immediately notice that manufacturers of formula in the UK are either actively infringing the regulation, or skating very close to the edge of it.

For example, the regulations prohibit the use of 'idealising images' on the packaging. Yet much of the infant formula available in the UK at the time of writing has representations of cute baby animals or cuddly toys on the label, or a representation of a parent holding their infant. Similarly, the regulations prohibit advertising that makes the brand the focus of the advert, rather than specific products, and that includes pictures or text which directly or indirectly relate or compare products to breastmilk. There have been many instances of advertising where these regulations have been ignored, and organisations including The Baby Feeding Law Group, First Steps Nutrition and Baby Milk Action collect examples and try to have the regulations enforced.

How do parents really make choices?

If we listen to parents describing how they chose the brand of infant formula they used, we can see that in many cases they did not have access to any of the information we have just discussed, either due to circumstances or because they did not realise that the information existed or might be important.

> *'When I had my first baby I knew I was going to formula feed and so I got some SMA in before she was born. I was fed on SMA, so were my brother and sisters – it's what my Mum said was best.'* Jemma, mum of four

> *'With my firstborn I wasn't given any choice! I woke from theatre to find he'd already been given Cow & Gate by bottle... when I had P I chose Cow & Gate because of previously having used that and not knowing any different! I honestly don't recall being given any advice*

by anyone... Cow & Gate seemed to be advertised everywhere so I naïvely thought it was the best!' Lucy, mum of three

'I tried expressing for the first time at 9pm one night and only got 30ml. I panicked and rushed to Asda for formula, thinking I mustn't have enough milk and that's why he cried every evening (never mind that he'd gained a pound above his birth weight in the first 10 days on breastmilk alone!). I was so anxious, sleep-deprived and generally (uncharacteristically) stupid that for a brief while I actually believed that "immunofortis" or whatever Aptamil claimed to contain, was a real thing'. Sarah, mum of two

'When I was told needed to top up, I was so disappointed – I had always planned to breastfeed. I felt really guilty like I had let my little boy down, so I chose the best on the market, the most expensive. When the nurse at the weighing clinic asked which one I had chosen she responded "Oh Aptamil, that's supposed to be the closest to breastmilk" so I thought I had done the right thing, made a good choice. She also told me I needn't feel guilty, that plenty of mothers chose to formula feed – but I hadn't asked to be excused, I had asked for help with getting breastfeeding established. I went home feeling angry, not reassured'. Stevie, first-time mum

'Ashamed now to say, I chose SMA mainly because that's what the hospital had in stock and then because the packaging looked the most "professional" when I was panicking. At hospital, I was told all formulas are the same and was put under a lot of pressure to make a decision immediately, when it wasn't something I'd ever

looked into as I was so sure I'd be breastfeeding.' Anna, mum of one

In Jemma's story on page 17, she made a decision based on a product her mother had used perhaps 20–30 years earlier. We know that the ingredients and composition of formula change all the time – so the product her mother used was actually a completely different type of milk with the same name.

If you have ever purchased infant formula, can you recall why you initially chose that brand and type? If you're thinking about choosing formula now, it can be worthwhile to look at some of your assumptions about branding, quality and health claims – at the very least, it might save you some money.

What are the different types of milks?

The baby aisle in any supermarket offers a baffling array of products. There are tubs of powder which need making up with recently boiled water, and bottles of 'ready to feed' milks. There are milks for different age groups, milks for babies who are 'hungrier' and there are milks which make claims about health benefits or are aimed at babies with health issues.

Most infant formulas are based on cows' milk, with lots of additional ingredients (just look at the list on a random tub!), but goats' milk and soy milk options are also available. Some of the products are labelled as suitable 'from birth', but these include products called 'first infant milk', 'comfort milk', 'hungry baby milk', 'partially hydrolysed', and 'lactose free'. We will cover these below.

Most standard milks in the UK are available in both powder and liquid 'ready to feed' form – so you have the choice of the less expensive one which needs making up in a clean sterilised bottle with very hot water, and then cooling before feeding to baby (see Chapter 2 for more on the 'how' and 'why' of making up milk from powder), or the far easier but more expensive pasteurised liquid in a ready-to use bottle which is already made up for you. Sometimes the liquid milks come in cartons, designed to be poured into clean sterilised bottles.

First infant milks are intended for babies who are being formula fed, or combination breast-and-formula fed, from birth until 12 months when they no longer require infant formula milk and can move on to unmodified whole cream cows' milk. There is no need to ever move your baby to anything other than 'first infant milk' except under instruction from a specialist to combat a particular health issue.

In the UK, first infant milks are *whey based*, which means that the protein ratio of whey to casein (two types of milk protein) favours whey. In the most common first infant milks, there are 60 parts whey to 40 parts casein, expressed as 60:40 whey:casein. (One product makes health claims about a ratio of 70:30 being closer to the profile of human milk, which is 80:20).

'Hungry baby' milk, by contrast, has a whey:casein ratio of 20:80 and so, in the words of one manufacturer, *'contains a special balance of milk protein designed to help your hungry baby feel more satisfied'*. It's important to point out that they also say *'if your bottle-fed little one has a bigger appetite and it's too early to introduce solid foods, infant milk for hungrier babies is a nutritionally complete breastmilk substitute...'*. In fact, hungry baby milks have exactly the same amount of calories, with slightly more carbohydrate and slightly less fat, as standard infant formula. So how do they 'fill your little one up for longer'? Simply because the protein balance takes longer to digest and causes slower gastric emptying, putting more strain on the digestive organs. Better to feed standard first infant milk in a responsive/baby-led way (see Chapter 3 for more on responsive feeding).

> *'There is no evidence that milks marketed for hungry babies offer any advantage, make babies full for longer, reduce waking or delay the introduction of solids. It is recommended that first infant formula is used throughout the first year of life if babies are not being breastfed. Milks marketed for hungry babies have more 'casein' than 'whey' in the protein mix, and casein is harder for babies to digest. An infant has a tiny tummy and needs to eat little and often, day and night, in the first few weeks and months.'*
>
> First Steps Nutrition Trust
>
> A Simple guide to Infant Milks, May 2021: page 7

Partially hydrolysed formula means that the cows' milk protein used to make the base of the product has been partially broken down: effectively some of the digestion has already taken place, with the aim of making the product less likely to cause stress to the infant's digestive system, provoke allergic reaction or trigger sensitivity to cows' milk protein. The evidence for this is not robust; if it were, perhaps all formula-fed infants would benefit from receiving partially hydrolysed milk. Recently, new milks have been brought out which seem to be using this as their selling point – however, we know that the more processed a milk is, the higher the levels of some by-products of processing, called advanced glycation end products (AGEs) about which there is some ongoing concern.

Lactose-free infant formula usually replaces the lactose in the milk with another sugar, typically glucose, for those babies who are suffering from lactose intolerance. The ones available in the chemist and supermarket are technically only 'very low lactose' and are suitable for formula-fed babies experiencing temporary lactose intolerance following some sort of gastric insult, such as a tummy bug. Lactose is important for brain growth and any use of these products should be very short term. They are not suitable for the approximately 1 in 45,000 babies who are born with a recessive congenital disorder known as galactosaemia. These babies would have prescription-only truly lactose-free milk while they are exclusively milk fed.

Formula milks with reduced lactose, and which are partially hydrolysed, are commonly known as ***comfort milks***, and different claims are made for them in different countries: in the UK they are marketed as being '*for the dietary management of colic and constipation*', while in other parts of the world they are '*to prevent or lessen cow's milk and other allergies in infants*' or '*for cramps and painful defecation*' or '*for easy digestion*'.

Some of the partially hydrolysed formula brands are marketed for use in preventing cows' milk protein allergy. These are known as ***hypoallergenic milks***, or ***HA***. The evidence for the overall efficacy of these milks is weak, and although they have been around for several years they have not proven popular. (See Chapter 6 for more.)

So-called ***A2 milks*** are made with milk from cows which naturally produce milk in which the protein is high in A2 beta-casein rather than being a mix of A1 and A2 as in standard milk. These have been sold in other countries and appear relatively popular, but are new to the UK, with no claims being made about why they are necessary or appropriate; indeed, there appears to be no evidence that there are any benefits. These milks will be more expensive as the cows' milk used to make them is less commonly available.

Anti-reflux milks are products sold off the shelf in the UK to manage babies' reflux and regurgitation. They contain either carob bean gum or rice starch as a thickener, which means the product has to be made up with cooler water and begins to thicken on mixing, thickening further in the heat of the stomach. The aim is to encourage the feed to stay down. The labels stress that these products should not be used in combination with antacids (such as omeprazole) or other feed thickeners (such as Gaviscon or Carobel). Finding the cause of the complaint is usually better than suppressing symptoms.

In 2004 the Chief Medical Officer issued a statement advising against the use of ***soy-based formula*** in infants even if they have cows' milk protein allergy, due to the presence of phyto-oestrogens, which may produce hormonal side effects: for example, fertility problems in adulthood. In addition there is an increased risk of allergic sensitisation to soya protein, which occurs in three out of five infants with cows' milk protein allergy. This is especially important in infants under six months of age and before the age of introduction of complementary foods, because milk is their only source of nutrition: soy formula should not be used under six months of age unless advised by a specialist. Soy formula is not hypoallergenic and should not be used in preference to an amino acid formula. Use of soy milk should be limited to exceptional circumstances, such as non-breastfed infants of vegan parents, or infants that do not tolerate other special infant formulas – and obviously, these parents should be advised of the risks so they can make an informed choice.

Goats' milk formula was allowed on the market for the first time in the UK in 2014, but is not widely used; indeed, the UK does not have a goat population large enough to provide for more than a very small number of formula-fed infants. The product is much more expensive than standard cows' milk formula. Some families whose babies have shown an allergy to cows' milk proteins have found success in eliminating the symptoms by switching to a goats' milk product, but we also know that a significant proportion of those babies with cows' milk protein allergy will also react to goats' milk proteins. Goats' milk-based standard formula is not available on prescription in the UK.

Follow-on milks are typically casein-based and aimed at babies who are over six months old and eating a good variety of family foods. Typically they contain more iron and sugar, and less fat, than first infant milks. They have no nutritional benefit over first infant milk, and are therefore not necessary, and their use is not recommended. However, they are marketed in very similar packaging to first infant milks, and, as they are not nutritionally complete (since they are aimed at babies who are getting the majority of their nutrition from their meals), most authorities urge caution when purchasing to avoid accidentally feeding follow-on milk to a younger baby who needs first infant formula.

On the 'older baby' shelves in the supermarkets you will find ***milks for older babies and toddlers***, which are labelled as 'growing up' or 'toddler' milks, and there are 'fussy eater' milks too. However, as first stage formula can be used up to and beyond 12 months of age, and from 12 months babies who are not breastfeeding and who do not exhibit allergic responses to dairy can be given normal full-fat cows' milk to drink, it is not necessary to buy these milks. They do not contain anything that your child cannot obtain from eating a range of standard family foods.

Just when you thought it couldn't get any more confusing, there are also milks for babies with digestive issues which are commonly issued on prescription by a GP, dietician or paediatrician, including 'extensively hydrolysed' and 'amino acid' formulas, and more rarely milks designed for babies who have been born very early or have other digestive issues. These are known as ***milks for special medical purposes***.

What's in formula?

There are very clear guidelines from the European Food Standards Agency (EFSA) on what can and cannot be in infant milks in Europe, and the levels which each product should have when ready to drink. Despite the UK's exit from the European Union, we have retained these guidelines – at least for now. There are minimum and maximum levels for the following ingredients:

Water
Protein
Fat
Essential fatty acids
Glycemic carbohydrates
Dietary fibre
Calcium
Sodium
Magnesium
Phosphorus
Chloride
Potassium
Iron
Copper
Chromium
Selenium
Iodine
Molybdenum
Manganese
Fluoride
Vitamins A, C, D, E, K, B1, B2, B6, B12
Niacin
Pantothenic acid
Biotin
Folate
Choline

There are maximum (but no minimum) levels of some toxic heavy metals, for example arsenic, mercury, tin, lead and cadmium.

Occasionally a news article pops up scaremongering about toxins and pollutants found in human milk, which may lead some to assume that formula feeding is safer. Samples from lactating women living in cities or near busy roads with car fumes, or near farms which use pesticides, or who spend time in homes or workplaces where there are perfumes, solvents or modern industrial chemicals, often contain small amounts of these toxins. But cows breathe the same air as we do, and eat grass which is rained on by our polluted clouds, and so you would expect to find the same toxins in formula milk.

> *'If all the crap is in breastmilk, surely it's in formula too? Or is it safely filtered out, or are all cows lentil-weaving groovy fruitarians, living in a hermetically sealed organic oxygen-rich biosphere?'* contributor to Netmums

What's crucial to understand is that although all formula milks are intended to meet the same standards, this does not mean that they are all the same, and so it's entirely possible that one sort of milk may suit a particular baby, while another does not.

What's not in formula?

Over the years, new ingredients have been added to formula once scientific evidence has shown that babies need them, and a cheap enough source of the ingredient has been found. Sometimes this happens quickly and most commercial formulas soon contain the new ingredients. At other times the process has taken longer.

For example, it was well known by those in the infant nutrition manufacturing industry in the late 1970s and 1980s that formula milks lacked the ingredients needed for optimal brain and visual development, but there was no global awareness of this among customers. It seems likely that this is why earlier introduction of solid foods was encouraged at this time. The missing items were ***omega-3 long-chain polyunsaturated fatty acids*** (LCPUFAs). Human milk contains a changing balance of 184 fatty acids, and attempts were made by manufacturing companies to add fatty acids from various sources to formula milks to increase levels of LCPUFAs. However, early trials of things like egg phospholipids in experimental formulas did not lead to their general introduction and – perhaps most worryingly – we don't know why. Perhaps it was too difficult to standardise the lipid composition from eggs, as it seems to vary with the hen's age. Perhaps they were tricky to source in sufficient quantity at acceptable cost. Perhaps they led to an increase in allergy in the longer term (there certainly is more hens' egg allergy recorded in our population now than at any time), but longer-term allergic response is apparently (from papers available to the public) not usually studied when changes to formula have been made.

There is a brand of milk on the market today which uses egg lipids, and to my knowledge the evidence for the long-term safety of these egg lipids in infant formula has not been widely studied. (For more information, see the work of First Steps Nutrition, or formula industry historian and allergy specialist Maureen Minchin.) This milk is given out in many hospitals which provide first milk for formula-fed babies, and it was put into the NHS supply chain and brought into hospitals without any information being provided about the change in composition. It's also at time of writing by far the most expensive standard milk on the market.

You will probably have heard that eating fish is good for the brain – oily fish contains omega-3 LCPUFAs – and in the 1990s formula milk manufacturing companies started adding it to their milks. Until the 1960s children were given cod liver oil supplements and often weaned at a few months of age onto vegetables with egg yolk mashed into them. Once formula milks started to claim to be 'complete nutrition', for example after the addition of A and D vitamins, paediatric authorities began to stress that supplementation was not necessary after cases of excess vitamin A making babies ill; here in the UK there was a worrying increase of hypercalcaemia (which is too much calcium in the blood).

There are many things which are present in breastmilk, which are not present in our 'breastmilk substitutes'. These include stem cells, enzymes, growth factors, hormones, anti-inflammatory compounds, live 'friendly' bacteria which colonise the gut and help with digestion and health, live viral fragments that trigger protective antibody responses and so on. And since the ingredients in human milk are human, they are very unlikely to trigger allergic responses in human babies.

What about added ingredients?

As we have seen, there are strict rules on what must and must not be in infant formula. There are maximum and/or minimum levels of many components, aimed at producing optimum growth and nutrition for the developing formula-fed infant, so far as our scientific knowledge and technological capabilities have made possible.

However, some brands include other ingredients which are not included in the ingredients list by law, but are 'allowed'. These include nucleotides (which appear in greater quantities and variety in human milk than in cows' milk, and are thought to be the reason for some of the differences in population risk of allergy and illness between cows' milk formula-fed babies and breastfed babies, although what they might 'do' is not yet understood), the long-chain polyunsaturated fatty acids or LCPs (known as DHA and ARA, or omega-6 and omega-3) as well as complex carbohydrates known as oligosaccharides or prebiotics (often referred to on packaging as GOS/FOS blend, for galacto-oligosaccharides and fructo-oligosaccharides, which just refers to where the carbohydrates have come from:

milk or fruit), which are intended to feed the infant's friendly gut bacteria.

In order to be allowed to add things into infant formula in the UK which are not specified in the existing legislation, the manufacturers need permission from the Food Standards Agency in the UK, which currently defers to the European Food Standards Agency (EFSA). The requirement is on the manufacturer to reassure EFSA that there are no detrimental effects of the ingredient, and there is a justifiable reason for including it. However, remember that:

1. All formula has to, by law via the Codex Alimentarius Global Standards, contain all the elements in specific amounts which are known to be essential for healthy infant growth and development, and
2. None of these essential components are allowed to be used to support claims made in advertising or on packaging about any advantage of that particular brand or product, and
3. Anything proven beyond doubt to be necessary to healthy infant growth and development will be quickly added to the list of elements required by the Codex Alimentarius Global Standards – but such proof takes time.

In the case of additional ingredients, therefore, these are not proven to be necessary, and arguably appear in the product simply so that claims about them can appear on the packaging, to promote the idea of the product's superiority. This only adds to confusion for purchasers.

Vegetarian/vegan/halal/kosher – and how they apply to formula

Vegetarian means the item does not contain any products which have required the death of an animal (including birds or fish) to produce them. Not all infant formula is vegetarian, as most contain ingredients such as rennet, which comes from animal stomachs, and oils from fish. There are only a few vegetarian infant formulas available in the UK, including Similac (available at time of writing only online) and Kendamil First and Kendamil Organic (available online or in some UK supermarkets).

Vegan means the item is made only from plant-based products, so it does not contain any animal milk, or fats from eggs. While we do have formula made from plant proteins (but see the discussion on the risks of soy formula earlier in this chapter), because the Vitamin D is sourced from sheep's wool there are no vegan infant formula milks for sale in the UK at present.

Halal means that the products have been certified halal (that is 'permissible' in Islamic law) by authorities in the Islamic faith, through an audit of practices and the specific methods of preparation – each manufacturer or each product might be separately certified. Some of the milks in the UK are halal, and they will generally say so on the tin – but because it changes depending on the factory in which it is produced, among other things, it's not possible to give an up-to-date list in this book.

Kosher means that a product is 'fit' or 'appropriate' for someone in the Jewish faith to consume, and has been effectively blessed or certified by a rabbi after assessment of the method of preparation. Some of the milks in the UK are kosher, and they will generally say so on the tin – but again, because it changes depending on the factory in which it is produced, among other things, we can't give a definitive list.

What about the cost?

In the UK, Aptamil is thought of as the most expensive brand, Cow & Gate as the least expensive and SMA and Hipp are closely matched in between. However, ongoing work from First Steps Nutrition Trust gives a breakdown of the recommended retail price of a tin, the volume of powder in the tin and the volume of powder required to make up a feed. The results are interesting. Additionally, in 2019 some new 'premium' and 'budget' brands were introduced onto the market, following the introduction of some supermarket own brands in previous years.

At time of writing (November 2021), these are the relevant recommended retail prices per tub for the main brands, arranged in price per 800g of powder, highest to lowest:

Aptamil ProFutura	£15.00
SMA Advanced	£15.00
Aptamil	£11.00
SMA Pro	£10.75
Hipp Organic	£10.50
Kendamil	£ 8.88
Cow & Gate	£ 8.69
SMA Little Steps	£ 8.20

This explains why some formula is security tagged: it's apparently one of the top 10 most pilfered items from UK supermarkets.

However, when we look at the amount of powder in a scoop (based on information obtained in November 2021), and the number of scoops needed to provide daily formula for a baby to drink (we used 30 ounces), this is the cost per week of powdered formula, highest to lowest:

Aptamil ProFutura	£18.11
SMA Advanced	£16.14
Aptamil	£13.28
SMA Pro	£12.13
Hipp Organic	£11.85
Cow & Gate	£10.27
Kendamil	£10.03
SMA Little Steps	£ 9.69

Next, we can look at the cost of the small bottles or larger Tetrapaks of ready-to-feed liquid formula – which is recommended for sick or vulnerable babies as it is pasteurised and does not have any bacterial contamination (in the USA, liquid feed is recommended for all formula-fed babies until at least a month of age), ordered here in daily cost of 920ml, highest to lowest:

Aptamil ProFutura	£5.06 (in 200ml bottles)
Aptamil	£4.37 (in 200ml bottles)
	£3.63 (in 1 litre cartons)
Hipp	£4.14 (in 200ml bottles)
Cow & Gate	£3.68 (in 200ml bottles)
	£3.22 (in 1 litre cartons)
SMA Pro	£3.68 (in 200ml bottles)
	£3.59 (in 1 litre cartons)
SMA Little Steps	£3.22 (in 200ml bottles)

There are other infant milks marketed for the UK including Nannycare and Kendamil Goat both currently (November 2021) £21 per 900g tub from supermarkets and online, Holle (another goats' milk based formula) at £14.50 for 400g, online, and Piccolo £14.99 for 800g, online.

In 2016 a product called Golden Country hit the shelves in shops such as Poundland, at just £1 for a 400g tin of infant formula, reportedly made in the UK. Many consumers instinctively react to the 'cheaper' products with comments such as '*Oh that's disgusting, what on earth is in that £1 milk?*', '*I would never feed my baby that, it must be bad for them*', and '*How could anyone put cost ahead of their baby's health?*'. But remember that the manufacturer of any infant formula milk product sold in the UK must do two things: firstly, they must declare their intention to sell the product to the government department responsible for infant milks and lodge a copy of the intended label for the outside of the product there with all required information correctly included on it, and secondly they must adhere to the EFSA composition requirements for the product inside. So formulas on sale in the UK all contain what is required by law in the appropriate amounts. This is vital information for consumers managing family budgets.

Finally, each product has a 'Feeding Guide' – an estimate of how much of each product would be used in 24 hours – on the packaging. This usually includes average amounts for babies aged 0–2 weeks, 2–4 weeks, 4–8 weeks, 8–12 weeks, 3–4 months, 4–5 months, 5–6 months and 7–12 months. Using this information we can come up with a cost for feeding a baby for a year assuming no wastage. Using November 2021's online costs for each product and the Feeding Guide from Nutricia Danone packaging, we get the following:

Aptamil Profutura	£789.96
SMA Advanced	£704.10
Aptamil	£579.31
SMA	£529.22
Hipp Organic	£516.91
Cow & Gate	£447.70
Kendamil	£437.60
SMA Little Steps	£422.46

There is a massive difference between the most expensive and least expensive. Comparing two products from the same manufacturer (Danone make Cow & Gate and all the Aptamil products, and Nestlé Nutrition make all the SMA products), which are made in the same factories, also gives us a clue about how much mark-up there might be on so-called 'premium products'.

Where is formula made?

At time of writing, there is no requirement for UK-marketed infant formula milks to state the country of origin of the ingredients, or the country of manufacture of the product. One company (Kendal Nutricare, which makes Kendamil) has called for this to be changed so that infant formula packaging must clearly state country of origin – perhaps this is because their product is made in the UK, which they hope will be seen as an advantage by consumers. Currently the main formulas sold in the UK are made in Europe, but they do not state this on their packaging – I had to contact the companies directly to find this information.

Conclusion

Much of the information in this chapter will be new to many readers. Has it changed your views about which formula is 'best'?

Knowledge about formula can help families, and their babies, and other babies yet to come. When we learn about risks, we have a better chance of avoiding and reducing them – such as in infant sleep, covered in Chapter 9, or in making up milk, covered in Chapter 5.

Without critically appraising the claims made by advertising and packaging we are left to decide whether to believe each piece of information as it is presented to us, and when we think about this, as most of the research about the ingredients in infant milks is done by or for the formula companies, it's hardly likely to be unbiased. Some of the research is done by paediatricians who genuinely want to know what is best, but this forms such a small part of the whole evidence base, in my experience, that it is easily lost. There will be more on this in Chapter 6.

All parents – in whatever circumstances they have made the decision to use formula milk – can benefit from knowing more about formula.

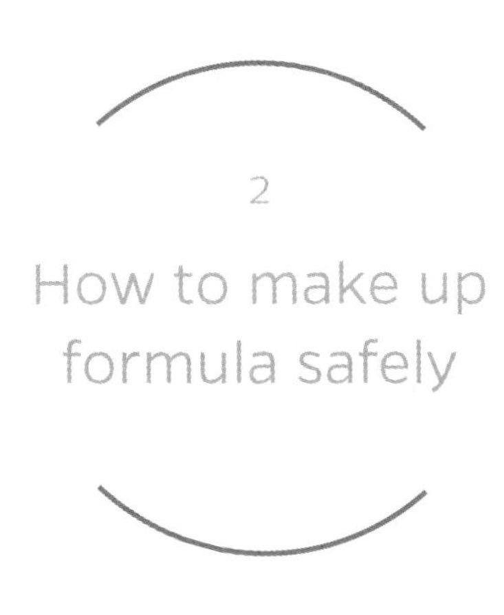

2
How to make up formula safely

If you have had a look at the packaging of standard infant formula you may have seen that above the instructions about washing hands/using boiling water/using the correct amount of powder/cooling the milk, there is the statement 'Because powdered milks are not sterile, failure to follow instructions may make your baby ill'. 'Not sterile' means that the product has not been heat-treated or prepared in a sterile environment, so contaminants can get into the powder before the tin is sealed. These contaminants can include insects or sometimes debris from the factory, as well as bacteria.

E.coli, *Salmonella* and *Cronobacter sakazakii* have all been found in powdered infant milks. While you may or may not have heard of these bacteria, or be aware of the effects of them on vulnerable babies, you are probably aware that milk is a fertile growth medium for bacteria, and warm milk even more so.

The World Health Organization, the UK governments, the NHS and the Royal College of Paediatrics and Child

Health all offer guidance on formula feeding (see www.who.int/foodsafety/publications/micro/PIF_Bottle_en.pdf for an example). This guidance attempts to strike a balance between the danger of not killing the pathogens in the powder if the water is not hot enough, and the fact that if the water is too hot it may destroy vital nutrients and the milk may be too hot when served, and risk scalding the baby's mouth.

Why can't we do what we used to do?

Until relatively recently (the advice in the NHS publication *The Pregnancy Book* changed in 1999), families making up bottles were advised to make up enough for 24 hours at one time and leave them standing – sometimes refrigerated but often not – until needed. This was partly because historically formula milks contained fewer ingredients and so there was less opportunity for bacterial contamination to occur in the mixing and assembly process than there is today, and partly because we did not really understand the consequences of bacterial contamination and the threat to our babies' immature guts.

> *'I know that the current guidelines say that you should make each bottle up fresh each time it is needed but when I was first doing bottles the guidelines were that you could keep them in the fridge for 24 hours and I've carried on doing this for my current baby with no ill effect, as have many other parents of second/third/fourth babies.'*
> *'I used to do that too, but DS had salmonella poisoning when he was five months old so I really wouldn't advise it. I know that the risk is extremely low, but I would not risk it. There was no other way that he could have caught salmonella other than from the formula – he was not yet weaned and no one else had it.'*
>
> exchange between parents on Mumsnet

Why can't powder be made sterile to keep babies safe?

Powdered infant formula is made by combining a number of pre-dried ingredients, which keeps costs down, and powders cannot be sterilised without making them unfit for consumption.

> Food production conditions are not sterile. They limit the number of microbes and contaminants allowed in the product rather than prohibit them. This means microbe levels that are considered not dangerous are allowed in the formula powder.
>
> …the very nature of the ingredients means that they cannot be sterile from the beginning. Therefore the only option would be to sterilise it after it is made.
>
> Powdered formula milk cannot be sterilised once made without either damaging the product or making it harmful to the consumer. The only ways of sterilising powders are:
>
> - Irradiation with gamma radiation
> - Dry heat sterilisation
> - Chemical sterilisation
>
> www.lifib.org.uk/why-isnt-powdered-milk-sterile

How do I reduce the risk of bacterial growth when making up powdered infant formula?

Following the instructions is key. It can help to assume that each batch *is* contaminated, perhaps before the packaging is opened and definitely after that, because air and dust and contaminants spread by fingers can get into the powder. The instructions in the Department of Health leaflet *A Parent's*

Guide to Bottle Feeding include 14 steps aimed at minimising the risk. These are detailed below with further explanation for each step. These instructions assume that the bottle and teat are already thoroughly cleaned and pre-sterilised for an infant under the age of 12 months (see below).

- Fill the kettle with at least 1 litre of fresh tap water from the cold tap. Don't use water that has been boiled before, as solutes (tiny particles of things other than the hydrogen and oxygen that make up water – H_2O) will stay in the water and some of the water will evaporate off on boiling, leaving the solutes (things like chlorine, metals and sodium) in a larger proportional concentration in the water.
- Boil the water. Then leave the water to cool in the kettle for no more than 30 minutes so that it remains at a temperature of at least 70°C.

A report published in 2009 on the bactericidal preparation of powdered infant formula found that water boiled and left for 30 minutes 'resulted in temperatures ranging from 46 to 74°C depending on the volume of water boiled'. Boiling 1 litre of water gave temperatures on average >70°C at 30 minutes. This report also found that some types of bacteria, such as *E. coli* and *Cronobacter*, were still able to grow at temperatures as high as 44°C.

- Clear, clean and disinfect the surface you are going to use so that it cannot contaminate the bottle.
- It's really important that you WASH YOUR HANDS, because our hands are one of the main ways that

germs are spread: harmful bacteria can be spread very easily from hands to food, work surfaces and equipment.

- If you are using a cold-water steriliser, shake off any excess solution from the bottle and the teat and, unless the manufacturer states that the product does not require rinsing, rinse the bottle with cooled boiled water from the kettle (not the tap).
- Using either fresh-washed hands or tongs provided by the steriliser manufacturer, pull the teat through the retaining ring. Keep the teat and cap on the upturned lid of the steriliser. Avoid putting them on the work surface because in spite of your efforts to clean and disinfect, this would increase the risk of contamination.
- Follow the manufacturer's instructions and pour the correct amount of water into the bottle. Double check that the water level is correct by holding it up to eye level before adding in the scoops of formula, because under- or over-diluting the milk can have negative consequences for babies (see Chapter 5).
- Loosely fill the clean, dry scoop with formula according to the manufacturer's instructions and level it off using either the flat edge of a clean, dry knife or the leveller provided. Powder might cling to a wet or dirty scoop or knife, and the powder might get contaminated by contact with things which are not clean. As above, under- or over-concentrating the milk can have negative consequences for babies.
- Holding the edge of the teat, put it on the bottle. Then screw the retaining ring onto the bottle tightly, so there are no leaks.
- Cover the teat with the cap and shake the bottle

until the powder is dissolved. Although shaking incorporates air into the liquid, you will be letting the bottle sit for a little while so the air will have time to rise up and escape the liquid again.
- Cool the formula so it is not too hot to drink. Do this by holding the bottom half of the bottle under cold running water. Move the bottle about under the tap to ensure even cooling. Make sure that the water does not get inside the bottle or into the cap covering the teat, because it might dilute the milk, and tap water is not sterile.
- Test the temperature of the infant formula on the inside of your wrist before giving it to your baby. It should be body temperature, which means it should feel warm or cool, but not hot.
- If there is any made-up infant formula left after a feed, throw it away. Warm or room-temperature infant formula is a great place for bacteria to multiply, and so any not neutralised by the near-boiling water, or which have come into the milk on contact with the baby's saliva, could have time to grow to worrying levels.

What else will I need?

It's really important that you are using accurately calibrated transparent bottles, with teats and teat covers, and you will also need something to clean them with, which should include a bottle brush and teat brush as well as detergent and clean water to rinse, and also sterilising equipment.

There are several ways in which you can sterilise your baby's feeding equipment, such as using a cold-water sterilising solution, steam sterilising, or sterilising by boiling. Remember to first wash your hands well with soap and water and clean the work surfaces with hot soapy water. As soon as possible after a feed, make sure that all milk traces are rinsed out with cold water, then before sterilising always clean the feeding bottle and teat in hot, soapy water using a clean bottle brush, and rinse all your equipment in clean, cold running water before sterilising (cold rather than hot water stops protein coagulation on the bottle).

When sterilising, first wash hands thoroughly, then clean and disinfect the surface where you will put together the bottle and teat. It is best to remove the bottles just before they are used. If you are not using the bottles immediately, then once sterilised and dry (drip dry from wet sterilising, or left in steam steriliser until dry) they need putting together fully with the teat and lid in place to prevent the inside of the sterilised bottle and the inside and outside of the teat from being contaminated. Remember not to dry them with a tea towel or similar as this will stop them being sterile.

But I never knew about all this!

This seems like a good time to say that if you have read the above and discovered that you have not been making up feeds as safely as possible, or perhaps you knew your family were not following the instructions, but did not know the reasons for the recommendations or the potential effects of any shortcuts, then you are perfectly entitled to feel shocked or guilty or have other feelings about this information. Whether you were not told, or were told but did not understand why it was important, or you understood why but found that practicality made it not the way you chose to sort out your bottles, what matters is simply that you move forward, doing the best you can with what you now know.

Sadly, good quality information about the absolute risk of gastric infection from not preparing powdered formula according to the recommendations is not available. That is not helpful for parents who want to make informed choices or the healthcare professionals who advise them. Presumably the data would be easy enough to gather, as babies with serious gastric episodes will access NHS services, so someone could collate some figures and extrapolate. But for now we do not have hard evidence to show the level of risk.

> *Early in this century, outbreaks of* Enterobacter sakazakii *among infants fed on powdered infant formula in Western Europe and the United States forced a rethinking of the cherished belief that artificial feeding is a very safe choice for infants in the developed world. Alarmed by these reports, the World Health Organization and the Food and Agriculture Organization convened an Expert Meeting in 2004 to determine the causes and again in 2006 to develop guidelines for reducing the risk to infants from intrinsic bacterial contamination in powdered infant formula. Reducing the frequency of contamination at the manufacturing level would eliminate about 80 per cent of the problem. Reconstituting the formula with water boiled and cooled to no less than 70°C is critical to destroy remaining bacteria. Arguments from the infant formula industry, some segments of the medical community, and some Western countries against this 'lethal step' trivialize the scope and severity of the problem and ignore clear scientific evidence.*
>
> Elizabeth Hormann,
> writing in *BIRTH* Vol 37: issue 1 March 2010

It is worth knowing that the risk of bacterial contamination from incorrect preparation of formula is immediate, not long term – so if you have been lucky, your child was never badly affected, and you may have got away with it! But knowing these facts may also explain some episodes of infant illness you could never understand.

Which bottles and teats are best?

There's a huge array of bottles and teats available, from 'anti colic' to 'bisphenol-A free', some are made from glass, some have wide necks or narrow necks, teats made from silicon or latex, teats made to look like a breast, bottles which claim to function like a breast, and many, many more. However, these claims are not necessarily evidence-based, so you can simply choose based on easy cleaning, cost and availability, if those are the things that you are most interested in.

IBCLC Philippa Pearson-Glaze has written a great piece comparing bottle teats and types for bottle-fed babies on her website (breastfeeding.support), which includes many of the types currently on sale in the UK. However, the article does omit the very wide-based teats which I feel are better for easing transition back and forth between breast and bottle, if that is your aim.

What else do I need to know about bottles?

We have stressed the importance of levelling the scoop and measuring the water correctly in the bottle to avoid over- or under-concentrating the milk, so it may alarm you to know that a study in Australia recently found that bottle calibrations are often 'out' by quite a bit – if you think about the fact that they are printed on to the outside of curved bottles, you can see how this can happen. It may be worth measuring your measures!

What about feeding in emergencies?

We don't like to think of ourselves as likely to fall victim to an emergency situation which might limit access to formula, water or power, but I can tell you that it happens all the time to people just like us, either from flooding or other bad weather making it impossible to leave the house or cutting off supplies, from fires or natural disasters locally, or even from something like being caught behind a serious road accident at feeding time.

> ***Infants who are not breastfed***
> *5.10 – In all emergencies, intervene to protect and support infants and children who are not breastfed to meet nutritional needs and minimise risks. The consequences of not breastfeeding are influenced by the age of the child (the youngest are most vulnerable); the infectious disease environment; access to assured supplies of appropriate breastmilk substitutes, fuel and feeding/cooking equipment; and WASH conditions.*
>
> International guidance on infant feeding in emergencies

In the flooding and resultant power cuts in my home county of Lancashire a few years back, which turned off the electricity and so closed the shops, some families walked miles to get to the hospital to beg at the doors of the maternity unit and children's ward for ready-to-feed milks. Helpful citizens were bringing in powdered milk, which was of course was not usable without clean running water or power. Some families were displaced from their homes for months due to flood damage.

Of course a baby who is being mixed-fed can be offered the breast more often in such circumstances, but clearly one of the major drawbacks of solely formula feeding is that we are reliant on our access to a product, to clean water and to power.

As we are often advised, as citizens, to be prepared for bad weather by putting snow shovels and blankets in our cars in winter, it's also worth thinking ahead about how you would manage with a formula-fed baby. You could perhaps keep a small supply of ready-to-feed milk available, and some water suitable for making up your baby's bottles (see below). Think about how you might access hot water for washing and sterilising, and how you might store milks that you have made up to transport.

Which water to use?

In the UK we now have pretty good standards for household water pipes, but if you live in an older house which might have metal pipes delivering the tap water, you might want to think about how to minimise the metals that make it into your baby's milk. Whether that is by buying water, or filtering your tap water, is up to you.

> *Bottled water is not recommended to make up a feed as it is not sterile and may contain too much salt (sodium) or sulphate. Water labelled as 'natural mineral water' may contain too much salt (sodium) or sulphate. If you have to use natural mineral water to make up a feed, check the label to make sure the sodium (also written as Na) level is less than 200 milligrams (mg) per litre, and the sulphate (also written as* SO_4*) content is not higher than 250 milligrams (mg) per litre. Like tap water, bottled water is not usually sterile, so if you have to use it you will still need to boil it before you prepare the feed.*
>
> NHS *Bottle Feeding* leaflet, 2015

Travelling away from home

When travelling, some families make up milk ahead of time and quickly cool it to transport in cool bags. The Department of Health guidance suggests that this is acceptable so long as the feed is prepared safely then cooled for at least one hour at the back of the fridge. You would then take it out of the fridge just before you leave and carry it in a cool bag with an ice pack, which would mean it could be stored for up to four hours. If you do not have an ice pack, or access to a fridge, then made-up infant formula must be used within two hours.

When reheating milk the Department of Health guidance advises against using a microwave as it can cause hot spots in the milk which can scald a baby's mouth. Many restaurants and play centres provide bottle warmers which heat the milk gently (but not quickly!).

Another way is to take pre-boiled water in a vacuum flask – which should stay above 70°C for several hours – and pre-measured formula, along with a pre-sterilised bottle. You can then make it up as needed, and cool it for baby to drink safely.

When travelling abroad, many parents worry whether the formula available to buy in other countries will be exactly the same as it is in the UK. For once, it may be worth ringing the company carelines for accurate information, because products with the same name can vary in composition. However, all infant milks in Europe are based on the same rules and regulations for composition, so they should be very similar.

One thing to check before you go, however, is whether the water in the tap in your room or lodgings is suitable for drinking, and whether there is a kettle. If the water is not drinking water, as is sometimes the case outside the UK, then you will need to find a bottled drinking water which meets the requirements outlined in the box opposite.

Also, think about how you will be cleaning and sterilising

your teats and bottles, and explore the possibility of investing in some small sterilising bags to take with you which can be purchased relatively cheaply online.

What about formula prep machines?

Over the years and across the world there have been many versions of formula preparation machines, some which you dump the can of powder into the top of like a ground coffee machine, most popular in the USA, and some which use capsules of powdered formula like a capsule coffee-maker – indeed the people behind the Nespresso machine also make BabyNes, which is popular in Europe. There doesn't seem to have been any formal appraisal of the safety of these sorts of machines, though during a peer supporter training course in 2017 the mothers I was working with provided some very interesting comments about cleaning and cost, and availability of the capsules, which is perhaps why in the UK we have one clear market leader in the preparation machine race.

Luckily, in the UK we also have First Steps Nutrition Trust, which evaluates the evidence for claims made about infant feeding products. This is what they have to say about the popular Perfect Prep machine:

> *'In the UK, while lots of new machines are coming on to the market in 2021, the only formula preparation machine currently available at high street retailers is the Tommee Tippee Perfect Prep™ Machine. This machine claims to "prepare a fresh bottle at just the right serving temperature within 2 minutes".*
>
> *The machine uses a two-step process to prepare the feed.*
>
> *In the first step the machine dispenses a 'hot shot' of water directly into the bottle. The user then has two minutes to add the [powdered infant formula], place the holding cap on the*

bottle, shake to mix and return the bottle to the machine.

In step 2, cold water is added by the machine to make up the selected feed volume to a comfortable temperature to feed immediately.

While research into the safety and efficacy of the Perfect Prep™ Machine has been carried out by the manufacturer, this is not currently in the public domain and the manufacturer has declined to release it for business competition reasons.'

Many parents have bought these machines and absolutely rave about them. Social media influencers often post about them. Tommee Tippee has steadily reduced the price so that more and more families have found them affordable. They even come in different colours.

An exposé revealed how hard it is to keep these machines clean, and also highlighted the fact that non-genuine filters can be purchased, which may not perform to the same standard (an internet search for 'perfect prep mould' will guide you to the story and claims made by parents).

However, of greater concern is whether the machine can prepare powdered formula milk up safely, as it does not neutralise the potential pathogens in the powder with an appropriate quantity of water at 70°C.

The Food Standards Agency made the following statement when asked about the safety of these formula machines in 2014:

'The issues we have with it are, although it states it dispenses a "hot shot" at 70°C to kill bacteria that potentially could be in the powder, the reality (if you watch the TT advert) is that this amount of hot water used is very small, and once this is dispensed into a cold bottle/cold powder the heat will be quickly lost (more so than when preparing a full bottle with cooled, boiled water to >70°C), so we would be interested to see whether

TT have done any validation to see what temperatures the hot shot/powder combo actually reaches (and whether this is enough to destroy any bacteria).The other issue, is that the rest of the bottle is then topped up with cold water, which TT state is filtered to remove impurities. Again, we would be interested to know whether it has been validated that the TT filter removes potential bacteria in the tap water (as this won't previously have been boiled). At present the Food Standards Agency would still advocate the use of our Best Practice Guidance, to use cooled, boiled water at >70°C to make up infant formula.'

from the First Steps Nutrition Trust document
Safety Advice on Milk Preparation Machines

This is what the same document says about using vacuum flasks to keep previously boiled water above 70°C to use to make up a bottle when out and about:

'The Department of Health recommend that the safest way to make up feeds from powdered infant formula (PIF) when away from home is to make the feed up freshly using a vacuum flask of boiled water. The boiling water should kill any bacteria present in the flask. The feed can then be made up in a sterilised feeding bottle using PIF pre-measured into a small, clean, dry container and the correct amount of boiled water from the vacuum flask. The Department of Health state that vacuum flasks, if full and securely sealed, will keep the water temperature above 70 °C for several hours. We have tested several typical vacuum flasks, with two volumes of water, over a period of between 1–3 hours, with the vacuum flasks warmed for 1 minute with boiling water before use and stored at an ambient temperature of about 19°C. We found the following average temperatures of water when the procedures were conducted three times, with each time test completed on a freshly stored batch of boiling water:

Amount of water in the bottle	*Temperature when boiling water first added to flask °C*	*Temp after 30 mins °C*	*Temp after 1hr °C*	*Temp after 2hrs °C*	*Temp after 3hrs °C*
Full flask: (approx. 17.5oz)	*92*	*90*	*90*	*86*	*76*
10oz	*92*	*80*	*74*	*72*	*66*
5oz	*92*	*72*	*70*	*64*	*58*

The 10oz flask of water was also tested at 2 hours and 30 minutes and the temperature had dropped to an average 68°C. This suggests that a minimum of 10oz of water should be carried in a flask, and that water should be used within 2 hours. Smaller amounts of 5oz will only remain at the correct temperature for about an hour. A full flask of water securely sealed as suggested by the Department of Health remains at >70°C for about 3 hours.'

There are plenty of other gadgets out there, seemingly a new one each time I look – but unless the manufacturers can show how they meet the guidelines for safe preparation or storage, it is not possible to make a fully informed choice to use them.

'The way I think is if it was that unsafe it wouldn't allowed to be on sale.' Mumsnet user, March 2017

If only this were true. I am appalled – and I imagine you are too – that products designed to feed our babies may not be as safe as we would expect.

Are there alternatives to powdered formula?

In the UK 'ready to feed' (RTF) infant milk/liquid infant formula is available.

> *'I used ready-made formula at £45 per week until my daughter went onto cows' milk, because after I stopped exclusively expressing for her, no one could tell me the safest way to make up her milk, in a way which was also practical. I heard one story from one health professional, another from the next, different versions from mummy friends, and something else again when I went to google. I was so scared I would poison her!'* Beverley, mum of one

More expensive by far, and available in individual bottles or larger cartons, RTF milk is pasteurised after being made and is sterile until opened. Parents also report that it seems thicker in consistency, and some health professionals wonder whether it may be more likely to cause softer poo, because the product has been ultra-heat-treated to pasteurise it, which may affect the sugars. There is no current evidence either way, on this.

Health Canada recommends that infants who are vulnerable to infection, such as those who are premature, have a low birth weight, or weakened immune systems, drink sterile liquid infant formula if they're not being breastfed or fed human milk. See the 'Best Start' publication entitled *Infant Formula What You Need To Know*, Ontario, 2017. Infant formulas available in Canada undergo a strict pre-market review process, which includes the assessment of data to show that the formula supports the normal growth and development of infants.

The US government's Centers for Disease Control and Prevention (CDC) says that all newborns should be on sterile liquid feeds and gives careful preparation recommendations for making up feeds from powder that is similar to the UK guidance. Unfortunately, it is not mandatory for the manufacturers to display this guidance on the tins or on their websites, and so they largely do not: most parents in the United States do not know about this issue. However see: www.cdc.gov/cronobacter/index.html

Because ready-to-feed milk carries much less risk of infection, it seems like the safest option, at least at first, for babies who are being fed formula. However, biofilms left on surfaces when complicated bottles and teats are insufficiently cleaned may still arise, and contamination from saliva backwashing into the bottle can occur, so the rule about using a feed within two hours of preparation still stands. If you are concerned, remember to swill the used bottle out with cold water straight after feeding, to reduce the amount of protein sticking to the surfaces.

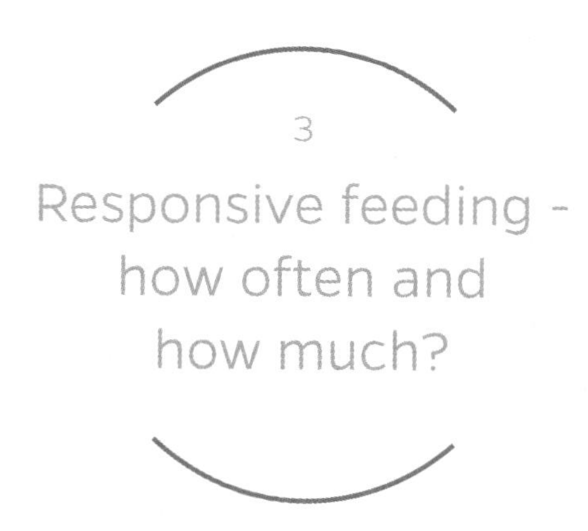

3 Responsive feeding - how often and how much?

Newborn babies have tiny stomachs, which are not yet fully formed (for example, the cells in a newborn's stomach walls are not quite joined up) and which are far from being sterile: they are already teeming with bacteria. These bacteria come from the amniotic fluid in their mother's womb, as well as from the birth canal, the mother's chest during skin-to-skin contact after birth, and being allowed to suckle at the breast. This colonisation by bacteria is a *good* thing, and it is what the baby's body is expecting. See *The Microbiome Effect: how your baby's birth affects their future health* by Toni Harman and Alex Wakeford for more about the microbiome, the filling-out of the cell structure of the newborn stomach wall and the initial seeding of the gut: here it's enough to say that although the newborn stomach is tiny, it has the potential to grow fast, because when food is in good supply our stomachs can temporarily stretch to accommodate more so that we can lay down extra fat stores for leaner times.

Of course, nowadays most of us rarely experience leaner times, except on purpose (when we go on a diet!), and when we do, our metabolism often slows so we can manage on less food. In this situation, with our swollen stomachs accommodating more than we need some of the time, actually a 'temporary' stretch often becomes a permanent stretch, and we feel hungrier more often than we should for our needs. This is thought to be one of the main reasons for obesity.

How does portion size for babies lead to obesity in later life?

This stomach stretching can begin in infancy if babies are overfed frequently, and it can lead to a tendency to be overweight if babies are fed when they are not hungry, and encouraged to finish the last of the bottle so we don't waste the expensive milk and so that they will go longer between feeds. Although formula feeding has been linked over the years with an increased risk of obesity in the infant/child/person when compared to human milk, we now know that this overfeeding risk when drinking too much from a bottle is likely to lead to obesity *regardless of what is in the bottle.* Scientists have found that early overfeeding can stretch the stomach in the early weeks and months of life, meaning that babies will then always crave more food than they really need in order to feel full.

Further, the association between being fed and feeling loved and cared for is an association we first make in childhood, and which might be stronger if we are fed large quantities (leading to feeling 'full' rather than just 'satisfied'). If attention and physical contact are otherwise infrequent, the association between a full tummy and what we perceive as 'love' may develop quite easily.

Doesn't what we eat matter too?

In addition to how much we are fed, and the way in which we are fed, in recent times it has become more and more apparent that *what* we are fed – that is what is *in* the milk which we receive as tiny infants – makes a huge difference.

Research into the so-called 'obesogenic' factors in formula milks has recently centred not just on calories per ounce compared to human milk, but also crucially on the amount of protein per ounce, as the higher protein levels found in artificial milks have been shown to be more likely to make babies put on weight and bulk than their breastfed counterparts. So compelling is this evidence that over the past decade or so protein levels in all standard infant formulas have been lowered.

In 2016 Nestlé SMA mounted a marketing campaign via press release featuring 'media doctor' Dr Ellie Cannon, whose website claims she is best known for a weekly column in the *Daily Mail*, and appearances on Sky News *Sunrise*. She was quoted in the press release (entitled '80% of mums surveyed did not know about the impact of too much protein on their baby's growth') talking about the changing profile of the type and quantity of protein in human milk over time as a baby ages. At the same time an SMA-branded video about protein was released online, and parenting bloggers were paid to review the 'new product' that SMA had released, which had a new, lower protein profile. This also drove traffic to the SMA Mums website, where there was more promotional material to read. Retailers across the country added old stocks of SMA to their clearance shelves in order to quickly dispose of the old formula with a 'protein level in excess of requirements'. Information received by healthcare workers from Nestlé presented a 'new improved' product, with a protein profile 'closer to breast milk' – but there was no apology for previous campaigns by Nestlé promoting old and now apparently outdated products, which would contribute to obesity, and which had also used the 'new improved' and 'closer to breastmilk' claims.

This reduction in the total amount of protein, together with a change in protein type (from casein-dominant to whey-dominant, and from beta-lactalbumin to alpha-lactalbumin to more closely mimic the type of protein in breastmilk rather than the protein in the cows' milk used to make the product) and fat structure (by altering the lipid profile and adding palmitic acid, to provide a poo consistency more like a breastfed baby) has been the crux of the claimed technological advances in recent years for standard formula. Recent research put forward by the formula industry shows that the tipping point for protein level is so important for a baby's appetite that if they are given milk with too little protein, they will simply demand more milk, so that in the end they get the same total amount of protein as in a higher-protein milk, but also far more carbohydrates and salts, and far more fluid, so stretching the stomach. The perfect balance in a breastmilk substitute is the smallest volume, with the lowest protein level, where all nutritional needs are met – so the stomach is not stretched. Thus, in recent years, we have seen the level of protein in infant milks drop to 11–12g per litre across the brands. This is, of course, good news for babies and parents. It does, however, raise questions about historic and current marketing claims, and also about what further research will reveal about other properties of formula milk in the future.

Reading confusing signals

Babies sometimes give signals that we can misread. Sometimes what we parents think is hunger is actually tiredness; sometimes what we think might be tiredness is actually a desire to be held, and sometimes what feels like a need to be constantly held is actually hunger. And around and around we go! New parents everywhere struggle to interpret their baby's cues. It can be helpful to understand what we know about how babies communicate their needs.

Babies are born with a few instinctual reflexes to get them through their first few moments and days of life:

- to take a breath once their whole face is in the air
- to push with their feet and pull with their hands towards the breast if placed safely on their mother's stomach or chest (videos online of 'the breast crawl' show how our newborn infants are not as helpless as we might think!)
- to 'root' towards anything that feels like it might have milk in if they are hungry
- to tip their head back and open their mouth wide if something makes contact with their chin and lips
- to suck on anything which touches the hard palate in the roof of their mouth
- to swallow any liquid which builds up in their mouth
- to stop sucking when they feel full, and to release the nipple

Some of these are 'use it or lose it' reflexes: if they are not rewarded with a response of food or attention or whatever was expected, the infant will become conditioned not to exhibit that reflex.

How do we know when our babies are hungry?

Some of the common early feeding cues which babies exhibit from birth include:

- licking lips and making 'lip smacking' noises
- opening and closing mouth
- sucking on lips, tongue, hands, fingers, toes, toys, clothing, or almost anything else

If these early 'cues' are rewarded with fairly immediate feeding then a baby will be happy and satiated, and they will continue to use the cues to communicate with their carers. If the feeding cues are never responded to, then the baby will soon stop wasting energy on producing them: sadly, this is part of how babies can be 'trained' to go longer between feeds, and never ask for feeds before they are offered them.

Active feeding cues might include:

- rooting around on the chest of whoever is carrying them
- fidgeting or squirming around a lot
- displaying discomfort or grunting
- trying to position for feeding, either by lying back or pulling on your clothes
- hitting you on the arm or chest repeatedly
- fussing or breathing fast

Later feeding cues will include:

- Moving head frantically from side to side
- Starting to cry

Why crying is *not* a feeding cue

It is important to note here that crying is *not* really a feeding cue: crying is a sign that we have failed to pick up on the earlier feeding cues, and the baby is now very unhappy, hoping to get us to notice them and realise we have missed their cues. Eventually, even a very hungry baby will cease crying to attract our attention and effectively 'shut down' to conserve energy. Sometimes parents and carers take this as a sign that the baby must have been tired and not hungry after all, particularly if the baby is being put into a routine for feeding, and this wasn't an allocated time for feeding. But when that infant *does* wake up, they will not act like a happy well-rested little person, but instead like a cranky 'hangry' baby, who shrieks and seems very high maintenance, because they went to sleep hungry and now they are *really* hungry, with no time to wait for us to figure out their feeding cues.

Some words about crying babies

> *'A baby's cry is precisely as serious as it sounds.'*
>
> Jean Liedloff, The Continuum Concept

As mentioned previously, some of the instincts babies are born with are 'use it or lose it' – a baby whose feeding cues are never rewarded with feeding, who is always left to cry, will soon stop exhibiting the feeding cues as they just use up valuable energy. If they find that they have to cry to be fed, then they will always do that. These babies may be seen as very high maintenance. However, if even their *cries* do not result in food, they will soon learn not to use up energy crying. They have learned that no one will respond. These babies often stop showing any emotions which are not rewarded with anything good, such as at sleep times if the parents are trying to 'sleep train', but sometimes babies of parents who have trouble with their own emotions can just start to suppress their emotions generally and have unrestrained outbursts now and again.

A happy baby is one whose needs are recognised and met as soon as possible, and who is held and comforted when they are unhappy.

Overfeeding

You may have heard health professionals say that 'you cannot overfeed a breastfed baby'. This is because breastfed babies do not usually take more milk than they need, for three reasons. Firstly, breastmilk changes during a feed from more carbohydrate-dense watery milk at the start, to denser, fattier milk towards the end. Secondly, a hormone in breastmilk called leptin makes the baby feel fuller as the feed progresses. Thirdly, the mother's milk ejection reflex responds differently at the start of the feed when the baby suckles quickly and rhythmically, than to the far slower suckles with long pauses that come later in the feed, when the baby may seem not to be feeding at all, and can seem like they are sleeping. All of these things mean that a breastfed baby slowly realises they're getting full, much as we adults do when eating a meal with breaks between the courses, or at a buffet where we have to keep getting up from our seat and going back to the table to get more. When bottle-feeding, whether there is breastmilk or formula in the bottle, things are different. The baby will – because of their instinct to suck if something touches their palate, and swallow if liquid is at the back of their mouth – often keep going until they have finished the bottle, if they are allowed to, and especially if they are encouraged to, to prevent wastage or to try to make the gap until the next feed as long as possible.

What we can offer babies to counteract this tendency, based on new best-practice guidance, is 'paced feeding' or 'responsive bottle feeding': this allows the baby more control over their feeding and encourages them to feed more slowly, taking breaks during the active parts of the feed rather than downing the bottle in double-quick time. For full descriptions of the method, see the article by Emma Pickett IBCLC on Essential Parent (search for 'responsive bottle feeding'), page 18 of the 2018 Department of Health/Start4Life *Guide to Bottle Feeding*, and the first side of a leaflet called 'Infant milk and responsive feeding' published by Unicef Baby Friendly and First Steps Nutrition Trust.

In brief, it's about allowing the baby to be in control and responding to their needs by feeding when they have given cues, keeping baby more upright than the traditional 'flat on back' position, allowing the baby to choose to take the offered teat, and with the bottle held at a more shallow angle so that gravity is not pushing milk into the baby's mouth. Then the adult would watch the child for signs that they need a break and pause the feed, perhaps actually lifting them upright to get any trapped gas out.

How much milk?

Many parents wonder how much milk they should offer at each feed, and how they will know when their baby has had enough milk in a day or a week. Should they follow the instructions on the packaging to judge what their baby will need? As you can see from the table, particularly the columns in bold (which have been added especially for this book, to show the actual volume the company anticipates a baby might require in 24 hours), it's not straightforward. It's often quite confusing!

Approx age	Approx weight	Number of level scoops	Quantity of water (ml)	Quantity of water (fl oz)	Feeds in 24 hours	**Total feed volume (ml)**	**Total feed volume (fl oz)**
Birth	3.5kg/7lb 5oz	3	90	3	6	**540**	**18**
2 weeks	4kg/8lb 8oz	4	120	4	6	**720**	**24**
2 months	5kg/11lb	6	180	6	6	**1080**	**36**
4 months	6.5kg/14lb 5oz	7	210	7	5	**1050**	**35**
6 months	7.5kg/16lb 5oz	8	240	8	4	**960**	**32**
7–12 mths	-	7	210	7	3	**630**	**21**

Typical 'Feeding Guide 0–12 months', adapted from formula milk packaging in UK, 2019

Looking at this table, is your three-day-old baby going to be able to take 540ml/18fl oz in one day – especially via six 90ml meals? Of course not. As we have established, babies' tummies are tiny and they are in proportion to their bodies: a rough guide is that everyone naturally has a stomach the size of the palm of their hand. Look at your baby's hand. New babies' stomachs do grow quite quickly – look online for pictures of 'infant stomach capacity' and you'll find pictures likening stomach sizes at different ages in the first days and weeks of a newborn baby's life to various fruit and nuts and so on, to give you an idea. Some healthcare professionals use so-called 'belly balls' to illustrate this too, but of course they can't be completely accurate as babies vary in size and build just as adults do.

Going back to the table, perhaps your baby is now 13 days old. Are they currently taking only six feeds a day, totalling 540ml in total? Well, gear up folks, because according to the packaging, tomorrow those same six feeds need to cram in 720ml as your baby hits the two-week milestone! And how many 13-week-old babies would be happy to go four hours between each feed? Clearly it's not possible, and nor is it desirable. The manufacturers themselves say these charts are a *guide.*

As you can see in the table from the two columns which are in bold type, the suggested volume of feeds in 24 hours actually *drops* to 1,050ml at 4–6 months, from 1,080ml at 2–4 months. Do babies actually need *less* milk as they get older? It seems counter-intuitive and it's just not the experience of families: babies at this age seem to be less satisfied and want more, and parents start to worry their babies are not getting enough from milk alone, and may need solid foods.

> *'Looking back now, smaller more regular feeds make much more sense, but we just went off the instructions to feed certain amounts every 4 hours!'* Amy, mum of two

Introducing food

Despite an EU ruling in 2016, many baby food manufacturers still label their jars as suitable from 4–6 months, causing some parents to believe that introducing solid foods at 17 weeks or so is an option. Further, some old-fashioned concepts are still in circulation, which suggest that babies' iron reserves will suddenly deplete at six months and so they'd better be on three square meals a day by then, and also that babies need to progress from sloppy purées to 'textured foods' and then lumps, before they can handle 'real food'. None of this is true. Puréeing foods *was* necessary, for those very young babies not yet able to sit unaided, without the fine motor skills to pick up food and get it to their mouth, whose gag reflexes and tongue function were not yet mature enough, at 17 weeks, to manoeuvre gummed food to the back of the mouth for swallowing. But now we have very clear evidence that healthy family foods should be introduced in the middle of baby's first year, from about six months, when they are showing signs of developmental readiness. These signs include sitting up unaided, grabbing for example a pea between finger and thumb, or perhaps a piece of chicken or a broccoli floret or carrot baton in their fist, getting the food to their mouth then having the co-ordination for chewing and then swallowing it. So we can skip the whole faff of preparing separate foods for a baby, the expense of buying jars and pouches of processed whatever, the messy spoons of mush which dribble down clothes, have to be choo-choo-trained or here-comes-the-big-aeroplaned into babies' mouths, scraped off their faces and re-presented, and just sit with them at the table and eat our own dinners! Phew.

More and more families are now hearing about the 'six-month rule' and the developmental signs of readiness – there's a great Department of Health Start4Life leaflet entitled *Building blocks for a better start in life* available on the NHS website or as a paper copy, which contains sections called 'No rush to mush' and 'Taste for life' (and also 'Sweet as they are' about the types of foods which might not be great as starter foods!), and which reiterates what I am saying here and presents the evidence base simply for everyone. Health visitors and other specialists in many areas do 'introduction of solid foods' visits at around four months – not so that they can tell families how to start giving solids, but so that they can encourage waiting until six months.

Professor Charlotte Wright, paediatrician and epidemiologist, on the introduction of complementary foods before babies reach six months:

The world over, parents view the starting of solids as evidence of their child maturing, developing, moving on, and because of this are tempted to start them early. It is really important to resist this assumption, the danger being that introducing solids early will reduce the child's intake of breastmilk, which is really all they need for the first six months. Introducing anything else before this age increases the child's risk of infection, with a number of UK cohort studies showing that exclusively breastfed infants are healthier than partially or non-breastfed babies.

I've personally been involved in UK studies where even in formula-feeding children, starting solids very early (before four months) increased the risk of health problems such as diarrhoea, so the WHO recommendation applies to all babies.

In 2003 around 95% of babies had started solids by four months (as recommended at the time). It was completely normalised. By 2010, that proportion dropped to around 30%, with the majority of parents starting their child on solids between five and six months.

There is a push, particularly from the formula industry, for the recommendation to be changed from six months back to four–six months. We've reviewed all of the challenges and found no evidence for them. One argument is that waiting till six months to introduce solids runs the risk of children not having enough to eat and particularly not enough iron, but it actually has been found to have no increased risk of adverse weight gain or iron deficiency anaemia.

Recently there has been some press coverage of discussion among academics, such as Mary Fewtrell and Gideon Lack, who believe that introducing food to the milk-fed infant sooner may improve sleep. Every parent could use more sleep, so the articles were shared widely. However, there is little evidence for the idea, as well as counter-evidence in the form of research carried out by the Department of Child Health at the University of Swansea, and there are no plans to alter the guidance.

So let's return to common sense: the calorific value of formula milk, which is loosely equivalent to the more variable human milk, is 67kcal per 100ml of liquid. 100ml of liquid takes up roughly the same amount of space in an infant's body as 100g of something else, although depending on the foodstuff the milk may be digested more quickly. Most babies who are given food before six months will start with puréed fruits and vegetables. As an example, 100g of boiled and puréed carrot would offer around one-third of that amount of calories, while displacing the milk. This clearly suggests that the infant might be more rather than less hungry once having food alongside their milk.

So what about the baby who is requiring more and more milk, over and above what the formula packaging suggests they 'should' have, and who is too young or not yet developmentally ready for solids? Some might suggest moving on to 'hungry baby' or 'follow-on' milks, but these are both casein-based products, and they offer no more energy or nutrition per fluid ounce, they simply make the baby's digestive system work harder and take longer to process them. Thus they can give the impression that the baby is fuller for longer, when in fact the baby may be getting less milk than they require. In addition, follow-on milks are not complete nutrition – they are designed for use alongside complementary foods, so there's an assumption that much of the baby's nutrition is coming from fresh fruit and vegetables, meat, fish and other good sources of protein. Looking again at the chart on p. 63, milk decreases to just three bottles a day from the time solids are established, with a total feed volume each day of just 630ml, or 428.4kcal, rather than the 693kcal from infant milk prior to introducing complementary foods. So for the hungry baby too young for foods, the best answer is to offer a little more of their usual infant milk, and to feed responsively.

Under- and over-concentrating feeds

Sometimes parents are tempted to add in an extra scoop of powder when making up formula, to help satisfy what seems like a hungry or fractious baby. Sometimes parents have not realised that the water goes in first and then the powder. Sometimes genuine mistakes are made when parents are exhausted.

> *'We were talking the other day in the staff room to a colleague whose wife has recently had their first baby, and he was telling us that he couldn't believe that we as a society hadn't come up with a more fool-proof way of making up bottles, because twice the previous night he'd forgotten how many scoops he'd added to the water, and had to throw the whole thing away and start again. Other colleagues were sympathising and making suggestions, sharing stories of foolish things they'd done when their babies were little, and reassuring him that they felt one or two scoops either way if he went with his 'best guess' wouldn't make much difference in the long term, though I didn't think that was true – I'm thinking that dehydration or malnutrition are pretty serious! But it's true that being a new parent is exhausting. Sleep deprivation is used as torture! It's no wonder new parents get confused and make mistakes. I'm dreading it…'* Phil, dad-to-be

However, this is another type of overfeeding that could have long-term consequences if it happens regularly, and should be avoided. Similarly it is possible to underfeed, both in terms of the overall volume of milk if too little is offered, and by spacing feeds too far apart. Watering down feeds, or putting in too little powder, will mean that the baby does not get enough calories, and over time will lead to faltering weight gain.

Should formula-fed babies have extra water?

While it's true that sometimes, in particularly hot weather, or if baby seems dehydrated or constipated, it makes sense to offer a slightly older (6 months+) formula-fed baby an occasional ounce or so of water no more than once or twice per day, what actually happens when we supplement milk feeds with water is that some of the milk in the baby's diet is replaced by water – they simply ask for less milk in that 24-hour period. This is a recognised trick for adults wanting to eat less to lose weight, but is not suitable for babies who need the right balance of fats and calories to grow and develop. So routinely giving babies large amounts of additional water is not recommended.

Adding other things to babies' milk

In Chapter 5 we cover some of the novel ingredients added to milks, medical supplements and thickeners used when babies are regurgitating a lot. In the past many families chose to add cereals to milk in bottles to thicken it or to try to fill their baby's tummy for longer: this is absolutely *not* recommended. A baby's immature digestive system cannot tolerate cereals given in this way, and even if there are no short-term observable problems, they may suffer from the damage done to the developing gut later in life.

Additionally, and thankfully almost unthinkably for most

young parents today, over the last few decades our parents and grandparents were told to add whisky or brandy to bottles to help babies sleep, were prescribed Phenergan (a sleeping medication) by doctors to give to babies to make them sleep, and were advised to dip dummies in honey to help pacify babies and space out feeds. It goes without saying that none of these practices are acceptable today, though you may still hear people talking about them.

How do we know if baby is getting 'enough'?

We talk about babies' needs increasing from nil to about 20 ounces (around 580ml) by the middle of week two of life, and then up to around 25 ounces (750ml) by the end of week two. This may then rise very slowly over the next 5–6 months, up to around 30 ounces (900ml) – but these are massive generalisations, and will vary from baby to baby. Most babies will require *roughly* 150–200ml of formula per kg of the baby's weight each day after around two weeks of age, until food is introduced at around six months.

Though it may be easier to judge the intake of a bottle-fed baby, how do we know if the baby is getting 'enough', for them? Well in the early days and weeks we can look at wees and poos, just like we would for a breastfed baby.

The Department of Health information talks about expecting a minimum of six wees and two poos per day for at least the first 4–6 weeks.

Formula-fed baby poo tends to be different to breastfed baby poo, with many mothers describing it as being like toothpaste squeezed from a tube; a different consistency and speed of transit than breastfed baby poo, which is likened to korma sauce and can come out in a stream. However, a minimum of two poos per day until baby is at least a few weeks old is still to be expected.

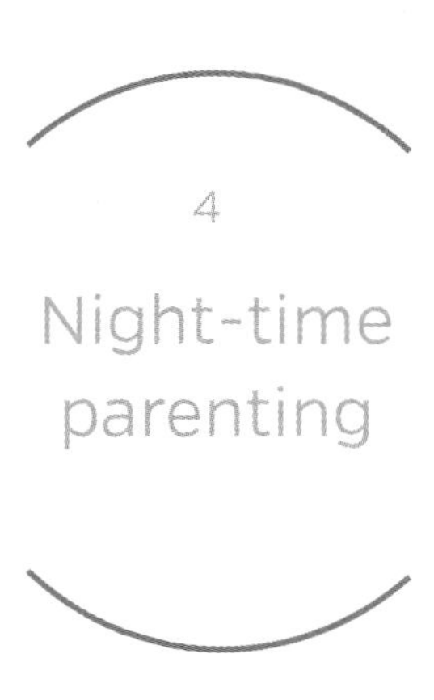

4 Night-time parenting

One of the most important issues for new parents is sleep. And we all know someone who seems to be getting more sleep than us, and we hear claims every day from those who say we would get more sleep if only we would do X or Y. But what we really need is the evidence.

It's normal and natural and biologically appropriate that new babies should be waking a lot and only seeming to nap a little between frequent feeds: their tummies are tiny and they don't know how to self-soothe. Formula or breast makes no difference to this biological fact when they are tiny; however, there are some useful bits of knowledge to share.

Do formula-fed babies sleep better? Why might it look like they do?

Formula-fed babies have roughly the same sleeping patterns in the first few weeks of life as breastfed babies, feeding day and night, with no distinguishable night and daytime sleep differences until around six weeks of age. However, studies show that after this formula-fed babies are able to take in more of the volume of milk they need in 24 hours during the day – or rather, not at night – meaning they 'slept through the night' sooner. It's worth noting that studies define 'sleeping through the night' as one continuous period of five hours from midnight to 5am. This may not be your personal definition!

So formula-fed *babies* appear to sleep for longer at night, but research has also shown that formula-feeding *mothers* get *less* sleep than their breastfeeding counterparts. Why might this be? One answer is that breastfeeding mothers who feed during the night release 'sleepy hormones' that help them to fall back to sleep quickly after feeds, and they do not necessarily need to be fully awake to breastfeed. Interestingly, breastfeeding mothers who have other people giving a bottle at night do not actually report longer sleep, although they may feel less isolated with shared baby care.

Strict feeding and sleeping regimes are less compatible with breastfeeding than bottle-feeding, so studies may reflect this: breastfeeding babies who naturally sleep well are less likely to be shifted to formula, while those that don't are more likely to be shifted to formula. It's entirely possible that the results of these comparison studies are skewed by complex factors.

For the baby, so-called 'opioid peptides' in standard cows' milk formula may induce sleep faster: although versions of these proteins are found in all mammal milks, human milk contains alpha-lactalbumin, whereas cows' milk is much higher in beta-lactalbumin, which is harder to digest. Essentially it is this combination of the type of opioid plus issues with slower digestibility, which means that new babies who are formula fed seem to sleep more easily.

Formula-fed infants have more REM (rapid eye movement) sleep than breastfed infants, who have more NREM (non-rapid eye movement) sleep. Formula-fed infants have been shown to have less arousability from active sleep between two and three months of age; which is partly why they appear to sleep better. However, this is also suggested as one of the reasons why SIDS is more common in formula-fed infants.

Higher protein levels in infant formula have been linked to an increase in the time spent in REM sleep – which in turn seems to affect calorie consumption and metabolism. Additionally, unlike breastmilk, formula doesn't contain tryptophan, a precursor to the chemical melatonin which we have as adults, which helps us establish our night and day, and makes us feel sleepy in the evening to help regulate our sleep.

Perhaps because of these sleep-promoting hormones, breastfed babies are more easily roused from active sleep – which may be a contributor to the breastfed infant's lower risk of SIDS, but also makes them more prone to night waking.

Overfilling baby's stomach

It is tempting to 'tank baby up' in the run-up to bedtime, in the belief that they will sleep for longer – but the converse may actually be true if a baby's tummy hurts from being overfull. No one advises a big meal before bedtime for adults!

We know that bottle-fed babies can be overfed, and that bottle-fed babies tend to drink more than breastfed babies, regardless of whether it's formula or expressed breastmilk in the bottle. It's well known that exclusively formula-fed babies will take larger volumes than are recommended, which is why we now advocate paced and responsive feeding (see Chapter 3). It's worth noting too, that to get enough nutrients, a baby needs to drink more formula (up to 300ml/day more around four months) than breastmilk, so those feeding breastmilk by bottle should not think they need to give as much as the formula can says is a normal intake. Another finding is that the earlier the baby begins formula feeding, the more likely they are to overfeed, so there's a higher risk of obesity both immediately and as the child grows.

It's not ideal to be stretching the tummy to accommodate larger feed volumes, just to try to obtain a little more sleep at night. And it usually doesn't work.

Coping with night feeds

Another hot topic is how to approach feeding at night: do you make up the feed before bedtime and take it up with you, risking bacterial overgrowth in the warm milk before baby drinks it, or do you risk an upset baby when they wake and you have to prepare a feed fresh?

Both approaches have major drawbacks. Perhaps the most feasible approach is either to use ready-to-feed milk at night, at room temperature and poured into the bottle, or decanted then warmed quickly in an electric bottle warmer kept in the bedroom, or to make up a feed with pre-measured powder and pre-heated water kept in a flask. It should be noted that this second option is the most frequently used in my experience, and while there is some risk of the water not being hot enough to neutralise bacteria in the powder, the bottle is fed to the baby immediately so there is little time for bacterial growth in the milk.

I have heard it suggested – and I categorically advise against it – that parents should over-concentrate the formula powder in the run up to sleep time, so that the baby is not hungry again so quickly. Over-concentrated formula places strain on infant kidneys, and makes babies thirsty! So-called 'goodnight milks' were on sale with a similar principle – they included added cereal: complex carbs which would take longer to be broken down in the infant's digestive system. Thankfully, as people become aware of the risks of early gluten exposure, these seem to have fallen out of favour in the UK, but still exist elsewhere.

Where should baby sleep?

The best source of information about safer sleep for babies in the UK is the Infant Sleep Lab at Durham University's Anthropology Department. Their website BASIS – the Baby Sleep Information Source – can be found at www.basisonline.org.uk.

Around the world, and throughout human history, babies have slept close to their mothers, during the day and during the night. For the first few months of life she provides warmth, safety, comfort and food – and until the advent of advanced technology babies simply could not survive without their mothers.

Nowadays we are able to keep babies alive, warm, fed, and safe, without their mothers' bodies. Cribs were constructed, formula was devised, incubators were invented, and over the past century products became central in infant care. How we incorporate babies into our 21st century world, and how we might adapt today's lifestyles to accommodate babies' needs, are not things we often think about – but perhaps we should. Where we expect, encourage, and enable babies to sleep is just one of these issues.

What a baby biologically 'expects', and what today's environments provide, can often be far apart.

Finding the right path through all the potential risks and hazards for babies in today's environment can seem like picking your way through a minefield.

Even when you have thought ahead and planned

carefully to avoid the known risks, how do you cope with a baby who suddenly won't or can't sleep in the proper place, in the approved way, at the appropriate time? How can you make the other options as safe as possible, and prevent yourself from doing something dangerous? What are the least risky next options?

From www.basisonline.org.uk

All official national guidelines emphasise similar points for reducing the risk of Sudden Infant Death Syndrome (SIDS) and Sudden Unexpected Death of an Infant (SUDI):

- Place your baby on their back to sleep, in a safe space with a firm flat mattress, in a room with you
- Do not smoke in pregnancy or let anyone smoke in the same room as your baby
- Do not share a bed with your baby if you have been drinking alcohol, taking drugs, are a smoker, or your baby was born prematurely
- Never sleep with your baby on a sofa or armchair
- Do not let your baby get too hot or too cold, and keep your baby's head uncovered
- Breastfeed your baby

In addition to the excellent work from BASIS, websites from NHS Choices and the Lullaby Trust provide detailed information about reducing the risk of SIDS.

Research shows that not being breastfed increases the risk of SIDS/SUDI, and families who are formula feeding need this knowledge so they can take it into account when they are making decisions about where and how the family sleeps.

To summarise, babies' sleep is a tricky issue, with the

balance of needs to be considered individually in each family, each night. Parents need convenient feeding choices, and babies need feeding as safely as possible. Babies need to eat during the night; parents need to sleep. The key is to strike a balance between risk minimisation and the meeting of everyone's needs.

> *'To get more sleep we had to reorganise our lives – I would go to bed without the baby at 9pm while his dad kept him downstairs and gave him his last feed at about 11pm. He'd then put the baby to sleep in the crib next to me and go to sleep himself in the spare room. I'd look after the baby during the night, then his dad would come in and take him away when he woke up at about 6am, before giving him back to me when he went to work at 7. This way I got a few hours' sleep without the baby and so did my husband. It wasn't enough – it never is! – but it got us through the first few weeks.'*
>
> Susan, first-time mum

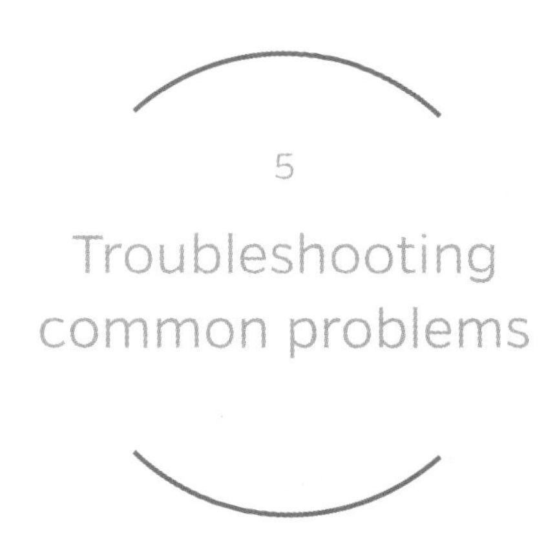

5 Troubleshooting common problems

Most feeding problems in young formula-fed babies can be eased by paying attention to the technique of feeding, the way the adult is making up the milk, or the type of milk the baby is receiving. However, there is a huge industry built around squeezing money from parents who really only want their baby to be happy and comfortable, and who will often spend huge amounts trying to solve perceived problems with their babies' feeding.

Below we discuss some of these feeding problems and how they might be addressed without resorting to medication or expensive gimmicks.

Some of the more common feeding problems in formula-fed babies include:

- baby clicking while feeding
- colicky symptoms/crying

- reflux symptoms – posseting and discomfort
- trapped wind
- sickness: posseting or more non-forceful regurgitation
- constipation – either infrequent stooling, or stools with drier consistency
- diarrhoea
- cows' milk protein allergy

Rarer problems include:

- faltering weight gain
- gastro-oesophageal reflux disease (GERD/GORD)
- galactosaemia

Common problems

Baby clicking while feeding

This distinctive 'click' implies that the baby is not maintaining a seal around the bottle teat, and so at the end of a suck the tongue is unlatching – perhaps allowing air to get in – and then the tongue is re-latching to form a seal so baby can suck again (this is sometimes referred to as the 'snap-back'). This is often tiring for a baby, and means they do not transfer milk from the bottle to their tummy effectively. It also probably means that they are taking in air with their feed, which can be painful and result in them bringing up some of their feed later. Some of the baby's stomach capacity is also taken up with air – which is not very nutritious! Babies who routinely click when they feed tend to gain weight more slowly, *or* spend a large part of their day feeding very slowly.

Often clicking is resolved simply by a) positioning the baby differently in the carer's arms, so that the baby is free to tip their head up and back, and to feed with their body held securely so that shoulders are above hips, so that they have a slightly tipped-back head while feeding, and b) positioning the bottle differently in the baby's mouth, with the teat directed up towards the soft palate at the back of the mouth, and the bottle pointed into baby's mouth up towards the top/back of the baby's head.

In this way the bottle teat will be far from the baby's nose, and the bottle itself will be nearer to the chin than the nose, so that the bottom lip and tongue are able to scoop around as much teat as possible to feed, reducing the click of the tongue's 'snap-back' as it unlatches and re-latches.

Discussions about optimal bottle-feeding often focus on the position of the baby, suggesting that keeping them more upright, rather than laying them flat, will give the baby more control and protect them from the 'drink or drown' feeling of milk pooling at the back of their mouth with gravity. Whatever technique you favour, it is important to avoid cradling the baby in the crook of the arm, because they will be too curled and not able to tip their head back or move away.

As I work with lots of families who are swapping between breast and bottle, I tend to suggest a more transferrable technique, keeping the bottle as horizontal as possible at first, with the base of teat opening the jaw wide and the end of teat up into the back of the palate to stimulate the baby's mouth in a way that is slightly more similar to breastfeeding. In this technique, baby's head and neck are supported by the middle finger and thumb either side of the jaw, and the shoulders are supported by the palm of the hand on the shoulder blades with the heel of the hand on the spine. The milk is kept in the teat by *slowly tilting baby and bottle back, together*, as the milk starts to be drained from the teat. Having the bottle more vertical, in a sub-optimal position, stimulates the mouth differently and allows the weight of more milk into the teat.

See the images, below.

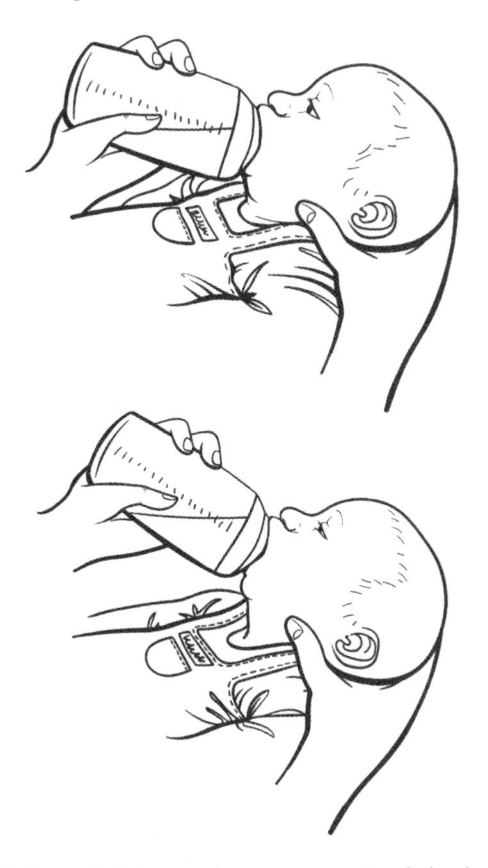

Bottle in baby's mouth in more-optimal (top) and less-optimal (below) positions.

Sometimes, however, clicking and slow milk transfer can result in an unhappy baby or one who is not gaining weight as expected. This might be due to a physical problem in the baby's mouth, for example an undiagnosed sub-mucosal cleft palate (where the bones in the roof of the mouth have not joined together properly while the baby was forming in utero), or, more likely, a tongue-tie in which the underside of the tongue is joined to the floor of the baby's mouth by a thin piece of tissue, which prevents the tongue from moving as it needs to, in order to be able to maintain a seal and so have good suction on the bottle, impairing the baby's ability to feed effectively.

Tongue-tie (medical name *ankyloglossia*) is an issue with the function of the mouth, present from birth, which reduces the mobility of the tongue and is caused by an unusually short or thick membrane (the 'lingual frenulum') connecting the underside of the tongue to the floor of the mouth. It can vary in degree of severity from mild cases characterised by a band of membrane under the surface of the skin at the rear of the base of the tongue, to complete ankyloglossia in which the tongue is tethered to the floor of the mouth.

Tongue-tie

If a bottle-fed baby has oral tissue tethering the tongue in some way, and this is negatively affecting feeding, and if the piece of tissue (called the frenulum) is thin enough and easy enough to reach, then an NHS maxillofacial surgeon, ENT (ear, nose and throat) specialist or a specially trained nurse can perform a small and fast procedure called a frenulotomy, frenotomy or sometimes a frenectomy. This is a simple 'snip' of that piece of tissue with special scissors, which can release the tongue to have the full range of movement it needs to be able to suck milk from the bottle and move the milk to the rear of the mouth, and to swallow while maintaining suction on the bottle teat.

In the UK we have access to this service through the NHS, and also via private practice. Unfortunately in some areas this service is only made available to babies who are not gaining weight as expected, or where they are breastfeeding and it is causing problems for the mother – this means that babies who do not meet these criteria may not be eligible to have the procedure done in their area on the NHS. The professional association for practitioners who perform frenotomies in the UK is the Association of Tongue-Tie Practitioners www.tongue-tie.org.uk, which provides a map directory of members on its website, although do note that the map only shows members of the professional association, and not all practitioners.

Sometimes parents are concerned about their babies seeming to have problems caused by high-arched palates, or by so-called 'lip ties'. If a baby has what appears to be a high-arched palate (where the bones of the roof of the mouth have met in a deep, steep-sided arch rather than a more shallow dome), this may be related to a tongue-tie which has tethered the tongue – or a part of the tongue – to the base of the mouth, and not allowed it the opportunity to help smooth off the palate as the baby was forming in utero, or when the baby was first born. Sometimes we see these high arches in babies who were born prematurely, as they also have not had time to smooth off the palate since the two bones were formed. In both these cases, a newborn baby can reshape the palate once they are free to move their tongue to smooth off/flatten out and widen the dome.

Lip ties are now increasingly referred to as part of a group of issues known as 'tethered oral tissue'. This term includes the obvious anterior (front) tongue-tie, the sneakier or less obvious posterior (rear) tongue-tie – both of which relate to the lingual (meaning tongue) frenulum, which is the bit of tissue between the underside of the tongue and the floor of the mouth – and lip ties or 'labial frenulum' (between gum and top lip), as well as cheek ties (sometimes called buccal ties). In fact there is no strong evidence that lip ties, no matter how big or how thick or how tight the labial frenulum, can negatively impact on a baby's feeding at all, where proper attention is paid to the position of baby/bottle, and technique of feeding, and after any other oral issues have been dealt with. Any jaw tightness, for example, resulting from the birth, or from having had a tongue-tie, can be treated by massage, infant cranial osteopathy, or infant chiropractic. Easy feeding is about the fit between the breast/bottle teat and the mouth it is going into, and there are many variables at work in both cases. NHS and NICE guidance does not support the division of lip ties as there is no evidence to suggest that it is helpful.

For further reading on tongue-tie, I suggest another book in this series, *Why Tongue-tie Matters*, by Sarah Oakley.

Babies with oral restrictions such as tongue-tie or high-arched palates can sometimes struggle to feed effectively from regular bottles, and parents spend lots of money trying to find the most effective bottle teat for their baby to use. Often bottle advertisements make wild claims about being closer to the experience of breastfeeding, but these claims are unsubstantiated. My experience, and that of my colleagues in the infant feeding world, is that for babies with a significant tongue-tie restricting feeding, the most effective teats are supple, narrow and long teats such as the Dr Brown's (which comes with its own issues, see Chapter 2 on the importance of thoroughly cleaning baby's bottles) or the Medela Special Needs Teat, which used to be called the Habermann Feeder. However, if you are planning to experiment with different teats, experience suggests that you may as well start at the cheaper end of the market. Babies are all different, and there's no sense investing huge sums of money when the pound shop stocks things you can try first that your baby is just as likely to be happy with. Ultimately, the type of teat that suits your child is down to the way they suck and their personal preference. The most important thing to check is that the product meets the British Standard BS 7368:1990 ('Specification for babies' elastomeric feeding bottle teats').

Colicky symptoms

Colic has been arbitrarily defined as 'paroxysmal crying', characterised by three hours or more of crying, for three days or more in a week, for three weeks or more, in an otherwise healthy infant, commencing from the third week of life. This was the definition given by Wessel's so-called 'rule of three' in 1954. This description was never very helpful, and means colic cannot be 'diagnosed' for three weeks, when in fact it can be present from soon after birth. It also doesn't describe or explain the baby's behaviour: if we think about it, a broken leg might result in the same symptoms, and indeed in the literature there are reports of babies whose 'colicky' symptoms turned out to be caused by hairs or threads (from clothing) wrapped around their toes, cutting off circulation, hidden away inside sleepsuits or socks! A more recent definition of infantile colic is 'spasmodic contraction of smooth muscle causing pain and discomfort', (Lawrence, 2015). Anyone familiar with the symptoms of a colicky infant will recognise this as suggestive of what is going on in that infant's gut: babies will often cry out, make fists, pull up their legs, go red in the face, arch their backs and thrash about in their carer's arms.

Colicky babies' crying can cause huge emotional stress and anxiety, or even depression for parents and carers.

As you will know if you've ever been unable to soothe a crying baby, the situation often reduces the adult to tears themselves, as they want so badly to stop the baby's obvious suffering. As hours of crying turn into days, anxious and exhausted parents turn to friends, family, health professionals, pharmacies and the internet for possible solutions, and at this point many fall prey to trying anything on offer. There are 'tried and trusted' (but not evidence-based) pharmacological and medical preparations, special devices, baby swings, swaddling blankets, massage therapies, homeopathy and sleep-training programmes... It's overwhelming for the whole family, and can be emotionally and financially draining too. Families I work with are understandably exhausted and desperately looking for an answer.

> *'You lay your hand against his skin and just rub his back. Blow into his ear. Press that baby up against your own skin and walk outside with him, where the night air will surround him, and moonlight fall on his face. Whistle, maybe. Dance. Hum. Pray.'*
>
> *How to calm a crying baby*, by Joyce Maynard

In my experience, 'colic' usually has an identifiable root cause. The baby's (and thus the parents') crying and suffering can be reduced by making changes in how the baby is cared for, handled or fed.

Some possible causes of intense infant discomfort include:

- *Infant anxiety.* Young infants can cry because they are alone and afraid in an unfamiliar environment, and crying is a major cause of air swallowing, while stress hormones affect gut function.
- *Trapped air.* Described later in this chapter, measures to prevent air swallowing as baby feeds make a big difference, as does learning how to help baby quickly and painlessly release any trapped gas which *is* in the stomach. Many of the remedies on sale which claim to reduce colic are targeted at this single cause.
- *Food allergy and hypersensitivity.* An allergic or intolerant reaction to one or more of the ingredients in the infant's milk. Identifying the trigger and changing the milk will remove the reaction – see the section later in this chapter on cows' milk protein allergy.
- *Parental anxiety and parenting techniques.* Sometimes, addressing the anxiety of the parent and trying just one thing at a time to soothe the baby (e.g. a simple sling that keeps baby upright against a warm body) or perhaps moving from a routine-led to a responsive feeding regime, or from controlled crying to attachment parenting techniques can make all the difference.
- *Microbial dysbiosis – an imbalance of the bacteria in the gut.* This can lead to fermentation of the infant's milk in their tummy, and associated discomfort.

Recent research suggests that 'too many' of certain sorts of bacteria and 'not enough' of others can cause a build-up of hydrogen and other gases from the bacteria fermenting milk in the gut. Evidence is emerging about which types of bacteria may be problematic, and how problems can be avoided in the first place. We know that the baby's stomach and intestinal flora and fauna – also sometimes called the microbiome – are affected by the type of birth they have (vaginal birth colonises the infant's gut very differently to caesarean delivery), whether they are able to have skin-to-skin immediately after birth so that they are exposed to microbes on their mother's skin, and how they are fed as newborns. Breastmilk contains hundreds of so-called 'friendly' bacteria, and a balance of around 200 so-far identified oligosaccharides (special carbohydrates which feed the 'friendly' bacteria), which balance the function of the infant gut as nature intended. Formula does not contain live bacteria – indeed, we go to great pains to kill all bacteria in the milk through the steps detailed in Chapter 2 – and only contains a few types of oligosaccharide synthesised from other foodstuffs. Some are now originally derived from human milk, but we have seen no evidence these are more effective. Formula also contains lots of free-floating iron, which feeds the so-called 'unfriendly' bacteria. More information can be found in *The Microbiome Effect: how your baby's birth affects their future health* by Toni Harman and Alex Wakeford, and *The Human Superorganism: How the Microbiome is Revolutionizing the Pursuit of a Healthy Life* by Rodney Dietert.

Chemical therapies for colicky symptoms

Simeticone (Infacol©) and dimeticone (Dentinox©) drops are often recommended to mothers. These products reduce the surface tension of gas bubbles in liquid, joining the bubbles of gas together, which supposedly aids dispersion as the baby can burp them up more easily. However, they have not been shown to be effective in reducing colicky symptoms.

Adding lactase enzymes (for example Colief©, Lact-Aid© or Co-Lactase©) to baby's milk has been suggested as a treatment for colic, to break down the milk sugar lactose into glucose and galactose. Randomised and blinded controlled studies, in which formula or expressed breastmilk had lactase or placebo added and were incubated for a period before being given to the baby, have failed to produce evidence for this approach. All families (including those who received the placebo) reported reduced crying over the study period. Possibly allowing formula to 'sit' refrigerated for some time before it was used allowed the air incorporated into it while mixing to rise and escape from the liquid. If necessary, a formula-fed baby can be fed a reduced-lactose or lactose-free formula in the short term, but comparative outcome studies are needed before recommending the long-term use in infant formula of carbohydrates that do not provide galactose, involved in normal brain growth. A degree of lactose intolerance in breastfed babies is often simply a transient effect of feeding issues, and can be readily managed if not caused by ongoing damage to the gut by, for example, milk protein intolerance.

Reflux symptoms

Reflux (proper name gastro-oesophageal reflux, or 'GOR') is a collection of symptoms sometimes described as a backward or return flow, or regurgitation. Symptoms include 'posset', non-forceful regurgitation, signs of stomach pain and gurgling sounds in the stomach. In its most severe form, 'GORD' or gastro-oesophageal reflux disease (sometimes known as 'GERD' because the US spells oesophageal without the first 'o') can present first as a baby with faltering growth, who resists feeding and also sometimes projectile vomits, spits up yellow liquid or what look like coffee grounds (actually bile and blood from stomach irritation), might have a hoarse cough or scream in pain, often when lying on their back, and not be able to be put down.

Reflux (so-called 'simple reflux' – not GORD) is a common issue of infancy, and although unpleasant, it is usually not a long-term problem. In fact, it can be a simple protective measure, as most babies will bring back excess intake.

There are many ways in which families and their infants can improve their quality of life and feeding, but the first-line treatment offered when the family seeks help from the GP is often alginate (such as Infant Gaviscon© or Carobel©), which is added to the infant's usual formula. The alginate often has the side-effect of causing constipation for the infant, as it thickens the matter in the stomach and continues into the gut where it hardens the stool: infants with constipation are often also prescribed lactulose to increase bowel motility.

There are also thickened milks, known as 'Anti Reflux' milks. In the UK the main manufacturers offer several options, although these are not approved by the Advisory Committee for Pharmaceutical Science: Danone's Aptamil and Cow & Gate brands both have versions at £14.00 per 800g/£11.50 per 800g, respectively; the Nestlé SMA version is £13.55 per 800g, and the Hipp version is £12.50 for 800g (Prices correct November 2021).

Thickened products, unlike regular formula, cannot be made up safely with 70°C water, because the liquid needs to be cool in the bottle and thicken in the stomach on contact with the heat of the body. This means the potential bacterial contamination of the product is not addressed by the method of preparation, so milks made this way must be used straight away and never stored, with all milk disposed of after one hour maximum – timed from powder hitting water, not from first touching the lips of the infant.

Chemical therapies for reflux symptoms

When thickening the milk doesn't work, as it often does not, the GP's next recourse is often to drugs like omeprazole, which is a proton pump inhibitor (PPI). PPIs block the action of histamine at the receptors of the parietal cells in the stomach. This decreases the production of stomach acid: their main action is a pronounced and long-lasting reduction of gastric acid production. These drugs may 'work' in the sense that reducing stomach acid reduces pain symptoms, but if it does not address the root cause of the issue then it's merely reducing the amount of stomach acid the infant has, and surely we need our gastric acid? It is not clear what the long-term effects of these drugs used in infancy might be. However, there are already concerns about the effect on the microbiome, on fat and mineral absorption and on bone density.

Silent reflux is described as reflux where the regurgitation is swallowed rather than exiting the mouth. It's not exactly 'silent', as babies may cry and show signs of distress, but they do not produce posset or 'spit up'. Symptoms may otherwise be identical to gastro-oesophageal reflux.

Guidance for dealing with reflux in infants

In the UK we are fortunate to have NICE guidance (guidelines produced by compiling systematic reviews of randomised controlled trials, plus expert opinion from specially selected guideline development groups) for many areas of care, which set out recommendations for best practice based on systematic reviews (to see which treatments might be most and least effective), economic modelling (to work out which treatments are most cost-effective) and expert opinion, to have first of all asked the right questions, and then to make the final recommendations. In 2015 NICE published guidance on treating Gastro-Oesophageal Reflux Disease, or 'GORD', in infants and children: online, search for 'Gastro-oesophageal reflux disease in children and young people: diagnosis and management' or www.nice.org.uk/guidance/ng1. This guidance clearly states that 'ordinary' GOR in infants *should not be treated with medicines*. This is because these medications are effectively using a sledgehammer to crack a nut: there are many ways to manage 'simple' reflux without medication, and we'll look at some of them here.

Often refluxy symptoms are actually the first sign of a food allergy, such as a cows' milk protein allergy, covered later in this chapter. Sometimes, however, it's simply that the baby is taking in too much milk in one go, or too much air *with* their milk, and regurgitation is the way they relieve the pressure in their gut. Trapped gas is covered later in this chapter too.

In the western world we seem culturally determined that babies should be lying in cots, so we keep them horizontal. This puts a lot of pressure on the valve which holds the milk in the stomach. Often simply holding the baby upright after feeds, or carrying them upright in a sling, can solve the 'spitting up' or regurgitation problem, and also reduce any pain baby may be feeling from liquid splashing up into the oesophagus. The following section on trapped wind explains how the sphincter at the top of the stomach works.

Sometimes, very rarely, in the early days, weeks and months of an infant's life, more serious issues like infantile seizures can be mistaken for reflux symptoms: infant feeding specialists might be the first people outside the family to see the baby feeding, and so spot something unusual in the fussy, jittery baby who is slow to gain weight and pulls away when feeding, crying out as if in pain. These seizures may also be characterised by 'arm circling' in the infant, and these infants are often overlooked at first, diagnosed with 'reflux' and parents sent away.

My message to you is that if you are worried, please keep asking for a further opinion for your child: your intuition about your child should never be dismissed, as so often parents turn out to be right about these things. And if you'd like to read more detail on reflux, do see another book in this series, *Why Infant Reflux Matters* by Carol Smyth.

Trapped wind

Typically when a baby has trapped wind they will show discomfort and possibly have a distended or 'tight' abdomen, which they communicate through high-pitched crying, sometimes flushing of the face, drawing up their knees, clenching their fists and arching their back.

Often trapped wind is caused by air being taken in and swallowed when the baby cries, or with the baby's milk – either from inside the bottle or, as they feed, via the sides of the mouth around the teat.

The simplest way for air to get in with milk is for the carer to introduce the bottle teat into baby's mouth full of air, and not tip the bottle up until it is in the baby's mouth and baby is sucking – so the first thing they receive for their efforts is 15ml of air! The way to resolve this is to ensure that the teat is already full of milk as it is introduced.

We have already seen that some babies cannot maintain a seal on the teat during the suck/swallow pattern because the movement of their tongue is restricted, and this may lead to air being taken in during the feed. Air intake can also be a problem if the bottle teat is being introduced into the middle of the baby's mouth, or if the baby's head is tipped forwards so that their spine is curved and their chin is near their chest.

To resolve this, the carer can attempt to alter their feeding technique so that baby's chest and neck are more extended up and back as baby feeds, and take care to introduce the teat to the baby's upper lip when the mouth is closed, encouraging baby to open their mouth and tip their head back so that the teat can go up on to the soft palate at the back of the roof of the mouth. The baby can then feed with the bottle resting more firmly on the bottom lip with the jaw nice and wide, with the teat of the bottle pointing up towards the top/back of baby's head. (See the figures on p 81)

Another cause of air intake can be gulping in panic if the flow of milk is too fast. One of my colleagues suggests including an exercise in antenatal classes in which one parent sits on the floor and feeds the other, who lies on the floor, with a bottle which almost pours into the mouth freely to illustrate how this must feel. A change in teat may be all that's needed to resolve this.

Another blindingly obvious but easily missed way in which air can get into the baby's stomach at the same time as the milk is if the parent or carer shakes the bottle to mix the powder with water, or when trying to cool a very hot bottle under a running tap or in a jug of iced water. Shaking the bottle can temporarily incorporate air into the milk, and there is not time for the air to rise out of the milk if the baby is fed straight away. The way to get around this is either to swirl the milk to mix it, to stir with a (clean and sterilised) spoon, or to make the bottle and then leave it to sit for 15-20 minutes before serving it to your baby.

Sometimes, as we saw earlier in the section on colic, the gas trapped in the stomach is not simply swallowed air, but gases generated by fermentation of the stomach contents. If your baby has trapped wind and measures to reduce the swallowing of air have not solved the problem, then what you need to know is how to release the trapped air in the stomach, which may otherwise cause pain both while it is in the stomach and once it has travelled down into the intestine.

Pharmacological preparations that claim to help 'get baby's wind up' have been discussed under 'colic' on p.88, but I believe that all parents can benefit from understanding how their baby's digestion works, so that they can encourage any trapped gas to exit the stomach 'upwards' as a burp, rather than 'downwards' through the guts to exit as a fart.

Winding your baby

Immediately after a feed, try this:

Hold baby upright against your chest, facing towards you with their head on your right shoulder and their bottom between your breasts/on your solar plexus. Keep baby in that position, with one of your hands lying gently on their back and your other hand supporting each buttock – thumb on one buttock and fingers on the other. The pressure and warmth on his abdomen will help him feel happier and more comfortable, the positioning of the hand on the buttocks means any gas or faeces can get out through the anus, and the position of the baby's digestive apparatus will ensure that the bubble of trapped gas is sitting directly under the sphincter when it opens to allow the gas up from the stomach into the oesophagus, and so out of the baby.

For more see the video on 'Wonky Winding'
on Shel Banks ILBC's YouTube channel

Sickness/vomiting/regurgitation of feed

Posset is very common – reports suggest 40% of babies bring back some milk, and it is often referred to as being a laundry issue rather than a medical issue. When the baby's sickness is 'just posset' – small amounts of curdled milk brought back up onto chin or bib or carer – or greater volumes of thinner milk which reappears via non-forceful regurgitation (no 'retching' associated with illness, and not forceful or 'projectile') then it's quite likely to be caused by either trapped air (see above) or some sort of food intolerance, which is covered in more detail later on. Both of these can be controlled – by modifying feeding technique or, in the case of cows' milk protein intolerance in a formula-fed infant, by changing to a prescription hypoallergenic milk to see if the symptoms ease or vanish. Ultimately if the baby is not distressed, and all other factors (for example weight gain, happy baby and so on) are fine, then a little posset is nothing to worry about.

Extensive posset/non-forceful regurgitation is one of the leading symptoms of infant reflux, which is covered below, and of allergy or intolerance to one or more of the ingredients in the milk the baby is receiving. This will generally manifest from birth, but it can take up to a month for the reaction to cause symptoms.

If your baby is suddenly starting to be sick and this is a new thing, then it's possible that they are suffering from some sort of virus or gastrointestinal bacterial infection. This may be infectious (e.g. a tummy bug) and the rest of the family may be suffering too, or in the case of a bacterial infection it's possible that the problem is actually the baby's milk, as infant formula powder has been found to contain bacteria such as *E. coli*, *Cronobacter sakazakii* and *Salmonella* which, if the formula has not been prepared or stored correctly, or if bottles and other feeding equipment have not been cleaned thoroughly, sterilised and dry stored before use, can build to levels which can make vulnerable new babies unwell. If a young baby starts to be unwell with vomiting, stop giving milk, as it can irritate the gut, but maintain fluids (very small quantities of cooled boiled water) and seek medical attention as soon as possible. Sadly, thousands of babies are hospitalised every year with dehydration following gastrointestinal infections. Dehydration can be dangerous in a young baby so urgent medical attention may be required: do make that phonecall to 111 or 999 if you have any concerns.

One question I am often asked is whether to offer more milk to a baby who has been sick recently; the answer to this is no, not if it is sickness, but perhaps yes, if it is actually simple regurgitation or reflux. Distinguishing between the two will give you the answer.

See Chapter 2 for more information on making up and using powdered milk to reduce the risk of bacterial contamination.

Constipation

This term is used in older children and adults to describe either infrequent stooling, or stools with a drier consistency than we would expect. In exclusively milk-fed babies, however, slowed frequency of stool which still has a 'korma sauce' consistency is *not* constipation. Babies under six weeks of age are expected to poo twice a day, every day, with these thin mustardy 'korma sauce'-like poos being at least the size of the palm of the baby's hand. A useful visual guide, with photos of nappies, is the NHS Scotland guide 'Off To A Good Start' under 'What's In A Nappy?', on pages 46-47 in the March 2020 version. If you're squeamish, an equally good visual guide is the Department of Health booklet 'Off To The Best Start' under 'How do I know that my baby is getting enough milk?' p.17 in the 24-page 2015 version, p.3 in the four-page 2018 version. A quick internet search for the names of these publications will find the latest versions. And, if you *really* enjoy baby poo comparison, you might want to have a look at the Facebook page 'Baby Poo Gallery', run by IBCLC Charlotte Treitl.

Causes of thicker or drier poo could include:

- over-concentration of formula bottles made up from powder, if there is too much powder for the volume of water in the bottle (see Chapter 2)
- adding rice or other cereal to the milk (which is not recommended)
- adding solids into the diet of a baby who is not yet developmentally ready for them (again, not recommended)
- adding alginate (e.g. Gaviscon or Carobel) to infant milk to manage reflux symptoms (see p.90)
- commencing solids but not offering water, so that baby gets dehydrated
- commencing solids which contain too much sodium (salt) so that baby gets dehydrated
- a food intolerance or allergy, for example to cows' milk protein (see below), soy, wheat or egg

The solution will depend on the cause – but is *never* going to be 'give them some fruit juice', as may be suggested by well-meaning friends and relatives. Fruit juice is not appropriate for a baby under 12 months. Mostly, constipation can be tackled by going back to basics and making up the milk just right. Sometimes it might involve a little bit of supplemental water. Consult a health professional if it doesn't clear up within a day or two, or if you are worried.

Diarrhoea

This term is used to describe stools with a very loose or watery consistency, possibly frothy, sometimes green or brown or yellow.

Causes could include:

- gastro-intestinal upset – virus, bacteria or food
- over-dilution of formula bottles made up from powder, if there is too little powder for the volume of water in the bottle
- adding solids into the diet of a baby who is not yet developmentally ready for them
- baby having medications, including antibiotics
- offering additional water to a milk-fed baby, which is not recommended
- a food intolerance or allergy, for example to cows' milk protein (see below), soy, fish or egg

Cows' Milk Protein Allergy

Cows' Milk Protein Allergy (CMPA) is the most common infant food allergy, affecting an estimated 1.9–4.9% of children worldwide, and an estimated 2–3% of UK children. This figure appears to be rising. It is an immune system response to one or both types of cows' milk proteins, the main groups of which are called casein and whey. Formula-fed babies develop CMPA after contact with the proteins in their cows' milk-based feed; exclusively breastfed babies develop CMPA as a result of milk proteins from products the mother has eaten transferring during pregnancy or through breastmilk. CMPA is very rare in exclusively breastfed babies whose family on both sides has no history of cows' milk allergy, but it can occur, even though the levels of cows' milk protein present in breastmilk are 100,000 times lower than those in cows' milk: the mechanism is not understood, but could be that the baby is reacting to the mother's antibody response to the protein in her system, rather than the protein itself. Babies who are mix-fed might develop the sensitivity from early introductions of cows' milk protein, say in hospital, and go on to be reactive to the protein (or antibodies) in their mother's milk too.

It is thought that the sensitivity to cows' milk protein is acquired in pregnancy, both through exposure via mum's diet, and by genetic disposition – basically the baby has a tendency to either being allergic or not being allergic, and if you think of it like a switch, that switch is either flicked to 'on' by experience and environment, or not switched to 'on' and left in the 'off' position. There are two types of CMPA, known as IgE-mediated and non-IgE-mediated. Babies may have one, or both.

Types of food allergy

There are two types of food allergy. The type depends on whether or not the allergic reaction is triggered by an antibody called immunoglobulin E (usually called IgE). These antibodies are the chemical signals that set off an acute (sudden) allergic reaction.

In an IgE-mediated food allergy, reactions usually happen within a few minutes of eating the food. Common symptoms are reddening of the skin, an itchy rash, and swelling of the lips, face or around the eyes. A rare but more serious reaction is anaphylaxis.

The other type of food allergy is called a non-IgE-mediated food allergy. This type of allergy is not caused by IgE antibodies – it is usually because of cell reactions in the immune system. Non-IgE-mediated reactions often appear several hours or days after the food is eaten and can cause symptoms over a longer period, such as eczema, diarrhoea, constipation and, in more severe cases, growth problems.

Sometimes children have a mixed reaction which causes both IgE and non-IgE symptoms and signs (for example, this happens in some children with cows' milk allergy).

IgE-mediated CMPA is the most common type, and the symptoms are more immediate. Symptoms which might be seen in infants include:

- a raised, itchy red rash: in some cases, skin is red and itchy, without a raised rash
- swelling of the face, mouth or other areas of the body
- nausea or vomiting
- abdominal pain or diarrhoea
- wheezing and coughing
- hay-fever-like symptoms, such as sneezing or itchy eyes

Non-IgE-mediated CMPA is less common. The symptoms of this type of allergy can take much longer to develop – sometimes up to several days or even weeks. Symptoms can be much less obvious and are sometimes thought of as being caused by something other than an allergy. Some symptoms which we might see in an infant would include:

- stools becoming much more frequent or loose (though not necessarily diarrhoea)
- constipation
- pain and sickness from reflux: stomach contents escaping upwards into the oesophagus
- blood and mucus in the stools
- redness around the anus, rectum and genitals
- unusually pale skin
- failure to grow at the expected rate
- excessive and inconsolable crying, even though baby is fed and clean: known as 'colic'

Of course, there could be other causes of all of these symptoms, for example, a less-than desirable feeding technique, eczema, *Candida* (thrush, a fungal infection), or viruses. Experienced and expert infant feeding support should be accessed to discount the more obvious potential causes, before looking for more complicated and rare ones: as a wise medic once said, 'When you hear hoofbeats, think of horses not zebras'. (This was said by Dr Theodore Woodward, who was a professor at the University of Maryland School of Medicine in the late 1940s, as an instruction to his medical students not to over-complicate their diagnostic technique.)

The NICE Clinical Knowledge Summary on CMPA says that if IgE-mediated CMPA is suspected given the clinical history, the infant should be referred to paediatric care for a skin-prick and/or specific IgE antibody blood test (previously known as a RAST test – and please note this test will not confirm non-IgE mediated CMPA) if there is:

- Faltering growth together with any gastrointestinal symptoms listed above
- One or more acute systemic reactions
- One or more severe delayed reactions
- Significant atopic eczema where multiple allergy is suspected
- Confirmed IgE-mediated food allergy and concurrent asthma/other allergies
- Persisting parental suspicion of food allergy despite a lack of supporting history

These tests may be performed in primary care if the expertise to conduct and interpret the test is available. The decision to perform a skin-prick test or a specific IgE antibody blood test in primary care should also be based on the results of the allergy-focused clinical history, and whether the test is available, suitable, safe, and acceptable to the child (or their parent or carer).

If your child ends up having these tests, the health professionals involved in their care should ensure that you are provided with appropriate information on:

- IgE-mediated cows' milk protein allergy, including information on what it is and the potential risk of a severe allergic reaction.
- The diagnostic process (skin-prick test and/or specific IgE antibody blood test).

Care of babies with confirmed IgE-mediated CMPA

CMPA is often seized on as a simple solution by doctors who can quickly prescribe a specialist milk, without a diagnosis (see Dr Chris van Tulleken's article in the *BMJ* about over-diagnosis and over-prescribing) – but the guidance tells us that formula-fed infants under six months of age who have been diagnosed with CMPA should be given a cows' milk protein-free diet until they are at least nine months of age, using a suitable extensively hydrolysed or possibly amino acid formula, given on prescription. They should also be referred to secondary care for diagnosis, dietetic support and advice on duration of treatment and the need for and timing of re-challenge to see if the intolerance has improved. Infants and children should also be referred to a paediatric consultant if growth/weight gain is not satisfactory on the special diet, or if symptoms are severe or there are other medical conditions present. If symptoms are severe, e.g. swelling or shortness of breath, future cows' milk protein challenges should be done under specialist supervision.

Although in this book we are focusing on the formula-fed

infant, as previously mentioned, breastfed infants can display symptoms too (though usually less severe) as some cows' milk proteins from the mother's diet can be found in breastmilk. Stopping breastfeeding in this case should be discouraged, with the breastfeeding mother following a dairy-free diet. Mothers should be advised to use a calcium and vitamin D supplement if they remain on a dairy-free diet long term and cannot be sure of getting the appropriate amount of calcium and vitamin D from their diet otherwise. A baby who is combination fed and reacts through breastmilk would require both their formula and their breastfeeding mother to be cows' milk protein free.

The diet of babies with suspected CMPA should be widened from 26 weeks as recommended, but referral to secondary care (paediatric dietician, paediatrician) is wise, to exclude other conditions and to access appropriate dietary advice. First Steps Nutrition Trust has excellent resources for suitable dairy-free foods for babies and young children at www.firststepsnutrition.org.

Because many infants get better at handling cows' milk proteins as they mature, a 're-trial' of dairy is recommended under 12 months, after the baby has begun to have complementary foods. For the breastfed baby, this would begin with the mother re-introducing milk into her own diet. One point to note is that babies who seem to have 'recovered' from their allergic symptoms (really they just get better at dealing with them as they mature) may relapse at times of illness or other physical stress, so keep an eye out for that.

If the specific IgE antibody blood test (RAST) is negative for CMPA, doctors might consider testing for allergy to other proteins including soy and egg. It's important to note that there are currently no validated tests to confirm non-IgE-mediated CMPA. The fact that there is no test means that this often goes undiagnosed.

Care of babies with non-IgE-mediated CMPA

Follow the advice for babies with IgE-mediated CMPA, but be aware that any cows' milk protein reintroduction should be managed carefully, in conjunction with a paediatric dietician, possibly with admission to hospital day care for oral challenge.

If the removal of dairy from the diet does not reduce symptoms, other potential allergens should be investigated as well/instead.

Multiple allergies

Babies with CMPA often also have allergies to other foods, for example other animal milks, soy, egg, fish and so on: once an allergy has been triggered, 'gut insult' can result in sensitivities to other allergens being triggered. As they begin to eat family foods, these allergies might include nuts, shellfish, gluten, sesame, 'nightshade vegetables' like potato, coconut or anything else. Pay close attention to symptoms and consult appropriate health professionals for support if needed.

Specialist formula for CMPA infants: used from birth to maximum 18 months

Extensively hydrolysed formulas available in the UK include (at time of writing): Nutramigen (Mead Johnson); Aptamil Pepti (Danone Nutricia) (contains some lactose, not suitable for infants with secondary lactose intolerance); SMA Althéra (Nestlé) and Alimentum (Abbott). Note: the Pepti and Althéra both contain lactose and instruct the user to make up safely with hot water to kill the pathogens; the other two require cooler water and so cannot be made up as per the safer preparation instructions.

Amino acid preparations in the UK include: Neocate Syneo and Neocate LCP (Danone Nutricia); Nutramigen AA (Mead

Johnson); SMA Alfamino (Nestlé).

These are the most commonly used products, but this list is not exhaustive. Infants with enterocolitis/proctitis with faltering growth, severe atopic dermatitis, or partially breastfed infants with symptoms during exclusive breastfeeding, are more likely to require amino acid-based formula.

These 'specialist formula' products are relatively expensive and usually available on NHS prescription since they are prescribed to infant residents. In the absence of independent comparative outcome data, it makes sense for the prescriber to begin with the least expensive product and work their way up the list only if the infant does not respond well to a product they have been prescribed, or perhaps to begin with the milks which can be made up with recently boiled water, and which still contain lactose.

In some areas of the UK, the burden of meeting the cost of a growing number of babies needing prescription specialist milks has led the local NHS Trusts to introduce a policy of only partial funding, or total non-funding, of these products. The prescriptions can still be issued, but the product will need to be partly or wholly paid for by the family. The expense to the family to date is roughly equivalent to the cost of standard infant formula. That seems fair, but it does emphasise the need for those with a family history of allergy to do all they can to achieve successful breastfeeding, especially those whose circumstances mean they cannot afford to purchase specialist infant formula. As much as I am certain that there are symptomatic infants who have not been identified as having CMPA, I am equally certain that the UK has an issue with the over-diagnosis of CMPA, leading to over-use of the prescription specialist milks. As the numbers of infants diagnosed with allergy rise, it is certain that costs will increase.

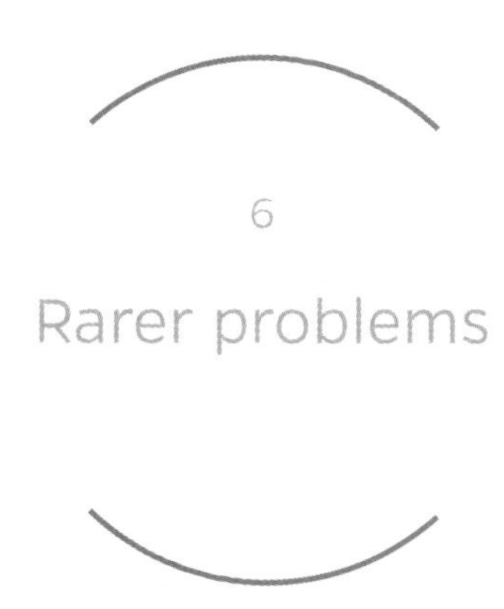

6
Rarer problems

Faltering growth

In the early days of feeding, bottle-fed babies are far less likely than their breastfed counterparts to have issues with faltering growth (which is when the baby does not make expected gains in weight and length). However, all babies can suffer from faltering growth and this is why there are regular weigh-ins and check-ups throughout the first months of life, as specified in the NICE Guideline on Postnatal Care (published in 2015 as Clinical Guideline 37 and updated in 2021 as NICE Guideline G194), and the NICE Guideline NG75 on Faltering Growth, published September 2017, which I helped to write. Faltering growth can be a sign that a baby is either not receiving enough milk or food, or is getting 'enough' milk or food but has some other issue affecting weight gain such as allergies or some sort of rare metabolic disorder. Identifying a problem as soon as possible is a good thing, as it can be an early warning sign of possible issues for that child later on. We know that good nutrition in the first years of life is a vital foundation for lifelong health and wellbeing, and that babies' brains and bodies grow incredibly quickly in the first year.

Broadly speaking, faltering growth would be considered if:

- Baby loses more than 10% of their birth weight in the first week of life
- Baby has not regained birth weight by the age of three weeks
- Baby consistently loses weight after first week of life
- Baby falls through centile lines on the UK WHO Growth Chart as follows:
  - More than 1 centile space if baby born below 9th centile
  - More than 2 centile spaces if baby born between 9th and 91st centiles
  - More than 3 centile spaces if baby born above 91st centile

For more information on faltering growth, including the standard of care expected for affected infants, please see NICE Guidance 75 at www.nice.org.uk/guidance/ng75.

Gastro-oesophageal reflux disease

NICE guidance NG1, 'Gastro-oesophageal reflux disease in children and young people: diagnosis and management', suggests that when an infant is experiencing more than simple reflux with 'spitting up', trapped intestinal gas and discomfort, some additional symptoms, for example faltering weight, blood in stool or in regurgitation, a persistent cough or hoarseness, or refusing feeds, might lead a GP to diagnose GORD and to medicate first with an alginate therapy, and if that was not effective then medications such as ranitidine or omeprazole which reduce acid production. *These will not remove the cause of the regurgitation, but will lessen the damage and pain associated with it.* Obviously the self-help techniques in the section on simple GOR in Chapter 5 should be tried first to rule out other causes.

Lactose intolerance and galactosaemia

Lactose intolerance and cows' milk protein allergy are not the same thing – and 'dairy' is not a cover-all term.

All milks made by mammals for their young contain a milk sugar called lactose – all so-called 'milkable' animals have roughly the same amount of lactose in their milk, around 3–4%, with humans having the highest percentage of any mammal at around 7% (thought to be to feed our larger-than-other-mammals' brains). Some primitive types of mammals, like the platypus, have a much smaller amount relative to the water and fats in the milk, and some large cold-water-dwelling mammals like seals, which have nutrient-dense, less-liquid milk, with pups getting their energy from the fat in their mothers' milk, have a far lower level of the sugar.

Because of this, all babies, whether human, cow, camel or kitten, are born expecting their mother's milk and so they have an enzyme called lactase, produced in their gut, which is there to help process this milk sugar, lactose, made by their mother. Without lactase we cannot use lactose in milk for energy and brain growth as our bodies cannot process it, typically resulting in bloating due to fermentation of the sugar by microbes, and diarrhoea. This basically describes what is meant by 'lactose intolerance'. There are three basic types of lactose-processing problems which humans can have.

Primary lactose intolerance is a congenital (inherited) inability to produce any one of the three enzymes needed to properly break down a sugar, galactose, produced when lactase (the enzyme) splits lactose (the sugar) into galactose and glucose. Glucose can be used immediately, but galactose has to be further processed. When not properly processed, it builds up in the blood (that's what the -aemia in galactosaemia means) and can damage organs including the brain. But this is a rare condition, and quickly diagnosed, as babies become very ill very soon after birth if they have this problem. The only treatment for galactosaemia is lifelong avoidance of lactose and galactose. Usually the baby is hospitalised in a large regional hospital where paediatricians specialise in managing galactosaemia. Neither breastfeeding nor mixed feeding is suitable for babies with galactosaemia, and even low-lactose formulas are not suitable. A special formula milk is used, and there are lifelong dietary consequences, as galactose exists in foods other than milk.

Almost all babies will produce the enzyme lactase. But some, at times, may not produce *enough* enzyme to digest the amount of lactose on offer. A secondary, temporary and transient (meaning it passes) lactase deficiency can be caused by any sort of damage to the gut, or 'gut insult'. Lactase is produced in the intestinal villi, finger-like projections of the gut lining, which recognise lactose and produce lactase to split it into glucose and galactose. If the villi are flattened by pressure or get damaged, lactase production drops temporarily. Gut insults might include a gastro-intestinal virus or bacterial infection (typically one which causes diarrhoea) or food poisoning, or might be a reaction to something as major as chemotherapy, or some other source of stress which causes the release of hormones that affect gut functioning. *Secondary, temporary lactose intolerance* can also be caused by allergens and chemicals which trigger gut reactions, such as those in cows' milk protein allergy.

Adult lactose intolerance can develop over time. The older body shuts down production of lactase, the enzyme which processes lactose, once the mammal is too old to be receiving its mother's milk. The majority of the population of the UK is unaffected by this type of lactase deficiency, as we have somehow evolved to continue producing lactase throughout our lives so that we can benefit from the additional calories and nutrients from domesticating dairy cows. Some populations, however, do still cease lactase production in later life, including the Chinese, Japanese and some central African and South Asian peoples. (Think about the food from your local Chinese takeaway – it typically has no dairy in it at all!). Generally this shut-down of lactase production takes place after the age of 10. Clearly no one's baby has this type of lactose processing problem.

Adult lactose intolerance is becoming more prevalent in once-tolerant western populations, and low-lactose or alternative milks have become widely available. In many cases people connect bloating and gassiness with drinking cows' milk, and fail to see this as a symptom of a secondary food intolerance, such as cows' milk protein-induced gut damage. While the noticeable bloating may be reduced by avoiding fresh milk, other symptoms may continue while sources of cows' milk protein remain in the diet. The emergence of secondary lactose intolerance in tolerant populations should be suspected as proof of ongoing gut insult.

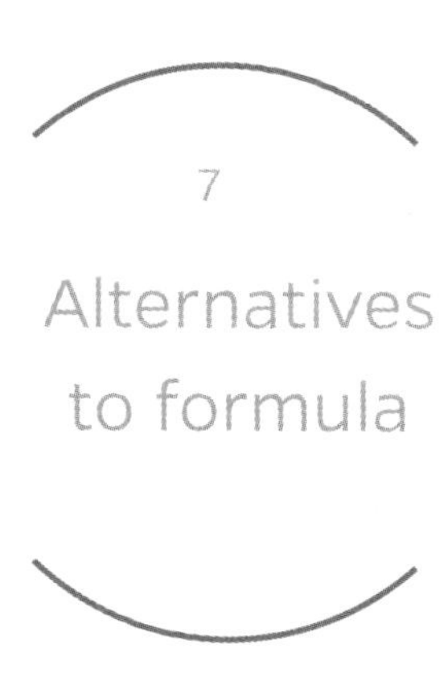

7 Alternatives to formula

In this chapter I'm going to discuss some things you might not have heard of, or ever considered. You might think that donor breastmilk, milk banking, peer-to-peer milk sharing, relactation and induced lactation aren't relevant to you – but it's my firm belief that they are part of the broad discussions about formula feeding that need to be had, and this chapter outlines why. We'll also look briefly at why homemade formula isn't a good option.

Sometimes families are advised to supplement a breastfed baby with formula without good cause, and without trying to improve the breastfeeding experience first. Reasons might include perceived delay of onset of lactation, faltering growth, prematurity, tongue-tie, illness – of baby or mum – or medication that the mother is taking. Or they might include reasons not to do with the health of the mother or baby, but the perceived difficulty of breastfeeding, the all-encompassing nature of being a new mother, or the desire of other family members to be more involved in the care of the infant.

Additionally, following the formula shortages in the shops at the start of, and indeed sporadically throughout the Covid-19 pandemic, it was very apparent that this information needed to be out in the public domain.

As discussed in earlier chapters, when we do not make confident and well-informed choices, we may come to regret them later as we discover new information, which can bring disappointment, anger, regret, sadness and guilt. Ensuring that feeding decisions are made with access to all the information needed, and the help of experienced and expert infant feeding specialists, is key to avoiding these negative consequences.

In the process of writing this book, and in the many years listening to parents talk about feeding their babies before it, I have been struck over and over again by how many of those writing or talking about infant feeding choices concentrate on not upsetting anyone's feelings, and worry about not inciting feelings of judgement. My view is that it is parents' absolute right to have the full range of impartial and unbiased evidence-based information upon which to make their choices – and this is often sadly lacking.

If a family is told by trusted medical professionals that their only choice is to formula feed, or they hear it repeatedly from different sources, then why would they not believe it? The truth, however, is that the vast majority of mothers who want to breastfeed their babies can be supported to do so fully and successfully, with access to the right information and expertise.

And for those mums who either are not able to access support, or are perhaps also facing other challenges elsewhere in life, or who simply choose not to breastfeed, for whatever reason (not my business to ask or judge), the truth is that there may be other choices than formula milk, and they are entitled to know about them.

'I was first told to use formula by a young midwife to fix the urates we observed in my newborn's nappy, and then a more experienced midwife challenged this after we had already started supplementing as instructed. Later, my community midwife told me to top up for weight gain, though my baby was gaining! I was not told about the top-up trap or the differences between formula and breastmilk in their composition and health outcomes. I wasn't signposted to breastfeeding support groups to get help. I know now that I made an uninformed decision that ended up costing me my sanity for months and plunging me into a darkness I never knew existed. It's almost five years and the pain is still raw; I am so angry that I wasn't informed about the risks of supplementing. I feel deceived and cheated out of making an informed choice in the best interest of my newborn and I, and our family, continue to pay for this in a variety of ways.'
Iyato, mum of two

Formula supplementation of the breastfeeding baby/ combination feeding

If breastfeeding isn't working out for your family, know that the decision to introduce formula feeds does not have to be all or nothing: some families plan to combination feed from the very beginning for various reasons, and countless more begin supplementing later on. A pattern of combination feeding can mean continuing to breastfeed or perhaps feed expressed milk at some times of the day, and feed formula at other times of the day. There may be benefits to keeping a foot in both camps.

The 'trick' to avoid the so-called 'top-up trap', if your intention is to combine breastfeeding and bottle-feeding, is to ensure that you are not increasing the volume of formula given each day. Choose the time of day when formula feeding will suit you best, and stick to it. Be aware of how your supply responds to longer feed intervals and, if need be, express rather than allow the breasts to get overfull, which tells the body to slow down production.

A baby who is bottle-feeding can become confused or frustrated at the breast. Bottle-feeding takes more energy, but depending on the teat and the size of the hole it can be *easier* than suckling at the breast. Responsive feeding, with the tipped-back head and frequent pauses described elsewhere in this book, is key.

As ever, it's just about getting the right information and support to make sure that we meet our goals and make informed choices, rather than being cornered into making uncomfortable decisions.

Banked donor human breastmilk

In addition to the baby's mother's own breastmilk, you may not be aware that breastmilk from other 'donor mums' is sometimes available to babies.

The UK has a network of milk banks – currently 16 dotted about our islands, which can provide donor human milk across Wales, Northern Ireland and Eire, Scotland and England. The milk banking association for our nations, UKAMB, was set up in 1997 and continues to go from strength to strength – not least because of a fundraising effort by a group of volunteer bikers known as the Relay Riders UK, which raised nearly £15,000 in 2018 to further the work of the organisation.

Milk banks typically supply donor milk for the very sickest and most vulnerable babies, in neonatal units across the land, to support their growth and development when the babies' own mothers are not able to make all the milk their babies need, or where there are some special situations. Milk can also be prescribed from these usually NHS-run milk banks for babies whose mothers are unable to provide their milk for a short period, for example where mum has to undergo a drug regimen such as chemotherapy, and so her milk would not be suitable for the baby. Sometimes NHS Trusts will procure milk for babies who are struggling to feed well enough from their mother and require supplementation, but this varies massively from area to area for the 14 milk banks which supply England and Wales, dependent on both the milk bank selected and the commissioning NHS Trust. It's more centrally funded in Scotland through the One Milk Bank for Scotland in Glasgow, which is funded on a pro rata basis for babies born all over Scotland, by all 14 Health Boards. In Ireland the situation is different again with the Human Milk Bank at Irvinestown providing milk to hospitals and communities on both sides of the border.

More information can be found at www.ukamb.org and via the NICE Guideline CG93 on Donor Milk Banking.

Peer-to-peer breastmilk sharing

In many countries around the world there is a market for donor milk, and it can be bought and sold online. In the UK, the UK Association for Milk Banking (UKAMB) statement on milk sharing sticks to discussion of milk donated for babies within the NHS system.

'The desire to help other mothers and their babies by donating breastmilk has been at the heart of milk banking for over a century and is truly inspiring. The numbers of milk banks and the numbers of infants receiving donated breastmilk is increasing throughout the world.

The National Institute for Health and Clinical Excellence (NICE) recommends that all donor milk administered in the NHS should be from milk banks that can demonstrate

> *adherence to the NICE guidelines on the operation of donor milk bank services. This includes the implementation of a quality control system followed by all staff and reviewed regularly. NICE also recommends that mothers should express and store their milk under hygienic conditions at home and follow their guidance to keep their milk free from unnecessary harms such as medicines, nicotine and alcohol.'*
>
> UKAMB statement on breastmilk sharing, 2016

Although we know that formula feeding can bring additional risks to the infant, peer-to-peer breastmilk sharing is not without risk either. Undoubtedly, the vast majority of mothers who express and collect their milk to donate to another family in need have the very best of intentions and will want to make all reasonable allowances to ensure that their milk is as safe and beneficial as possible to the recipient infant.

However, there is always an element of the unknown, even when we are dealing with close friends or family members, never mind other methods of sourcing donor milk. Sometimes the potential donor may be taking herbal or pharmaceutical preparations which could pass into milk and might cause harm to the recipient baby. And of course, while we can administer questionnaires to the donors to rule out those with various pre-existing conditions in which infection might be transmitted through the milk, sometimes the potential donor may not even know that they are affected. And milk which has not been collected or stored correctly might contain harmful pathogens, which is why milk banks rigorously screen both mothers and milk before sending milk out to our sickest babies.

A team of researchers from one of the United States' largest paediatric hospitals, based in Ohio, has conducted a number of studies on donor breastmilk sourced and paid for via the internet and shipped across the country to a PO box in Ohio, versus donor breastmilk samples obtained from a milk bank, to test the bacterial and microbial safety of the donor milk. They concluded:

> *'Human milk purchased via the Internet exhibited high overall bacterial growth and frequent contamination with pathogenic bacteria, reflecting poor collection, storage, or shipping practices. Infants consuming this milk are at risk for negative outcomes, particularly if born preterm or are medically compromised.'*

The researchers went on to state that 'Increased use of lactation support services may begin to address the milk supply gap for women who want to feed their child human milk but cannot meet his or her needs.'

It's important to note, however, that the addition of money into the arrangement will almost always alter the dynamic of the act of donation – it is no longer being freely given, and there's more motivation to increase the amount produced, even at the expense of a vulnerable infant.

The BBC reported in 2015 that breastmilk bought online (a reporter posed as the father of a six-month-old baby and bought milk from 12 mothers across the country) carried more bacteria than the milk banks in the UK typically find in donations. The 12 purchases were analysed by microbiologists at Coventry University, who discovered that a third of the samples (four) contained *E. coli*, two contained *Candida* (thrush) and one contained *Pseudomonas aeruginosa* (a nasty bacteria responsible for all sorts of infections).

Dr Sarah Steele, from Queen Mary University of London, told the BBC reporters that parents have *'heard the message breast is best, which is absolutely the case but this is stuff bought off the internet... you don't know the seller, you don't know how they've been storing it, you don't know what it contains and, more pertinently, they're often doing this for profit and that poses the risk that they may tamper with it, water it down, be it with water, formula, cow's milk or soya milk'.*

If you are interested in reading more about peer-to-peer donor milk sharing, there are plenty of well-evidenced and well-written articles online, but you could do worse than start with *Milk sharing: from private practice to public pursuit*, by James E. Akre, Karleen D. Gribble and Maureen Minchin.

Ways to responsibly source donor milk for babies

Globally there are a couple of networks that connect breastmilk donors with hopeful recipients: 'Eats on Feets' and 'Human Milk for Human Babies' (or 'HM4HB').

At time of writing, the UK HM4HB network is very clear that it is not responsible for making matches or for the milk itself, but it does go to great lengths to spell out how users of donor milk sourced via their pages can best reduce the risks inherent in using other mothers' milk.

The FAQ section explores how potential recipients can provide the safest possible milk, including getting full disclosure from the donor mother about her health and other circumstances including medications, alcohol and drug use, and what routine screening she has already had, including asking to see copies of antenatal test results for things like HIV, hepatitis B and C, syphilis, HTLV, cytomegalovirus (CMV) and tuberculosis.

Another option discussed is a low-tech version of home pasteurisation: flash heating, or HTST (high temperature short time) processing – which was initially designed to support mothers with HIV in developing countries to treat their own milk before giving it to their babies.

HM4HB also refers to standard guidance on appropriate storage of expressed breastmilk, standard guidance on reducing contamination via washing hands, cleaning and sterilising pumps and storage vessels, and on hand expression – which reduces the risk of contamination.

Additionally, where donors may be taking medications, HM4HB UK also signposts to the fantastic Drugs in Breastmilk information from expert lactation pharmacist Dr Wendy Jones and colleagues. This is available via the Breastfeeding Network website and Facebook page, as well as in her books – including *Why Mothers' Medication Matters* in this series.

Ultimately, mothers have been sharing their milk, wet-nursing and so on, since time began, and it is likely that this will continue with or without milk banks, regulation or scare stories on the internet. What is going to be vital is the provision of robust evidence and information so that, as with any other decision about their baby's health, mothers who are considering sharing milk informally can weigh up the risk versus benefit to those babies. They can take any measures they feel are appropriate to assess the safety of the milk they are considering using (which might include a donor information questionnaire, blood tests, and so on), but there are no guarantees. That being said, the same is also true of formula feeding.

Providing breastmilk via relactation or induced lactation

Relactation is the act of lactating again, sometimes after having birthed and stopped breastfeeding, while 'induced lactation' is lactation without having given birth. Increasingly mothers whose babies are born via a surrogate, or who are the non-gestational mother in a same-sex relationship, are choosing to lactate to feed their babies, at least in part – and with support and the right information it is totally achievable for many. Relactation is easier than inducing lactation without ever having birthed, because the pregnancy hormones have already created glandular tissue in the breasts.

If you have been formula feeding and want to return to breastfeeding, either in full or in part, or if you are interested in learning more simply because bodies are amazing things, there is plenty of information available. Take a look at the Association of Breastfeeding Mothers or Australian Breastfeeding Association websites to start with: type 'ABM relactation' and 'ABA relactation' into a search engine and you will find their information. If you're considering either approach yourself, I'd recommend finding good quality infant feeding support in your area.

> *'As a first time mum who didn't understand breastfeeding and had moved over to formula at two weeks, I felt I'd failed; when I learned about relactation and was able to rebuild a breastmilk supply, it was transformative for me as a mother. It was hard, intense work but deeply satisfying to see my milk supply return.*
>
> *The experience was so important for me that I pursued a career in breastfeeding support and then qualified as an IBCLC in 2018, with my main goal being to offer the warm, empathic and patient support I had needed when I was struggling with breastfeeding.'* Lucy, mum of two

Feeding from other than bottles

If you plan to mix-feed, you may prefer to avoid bottles. In many parents' and practitioners' experience, babies' ability to suckle at the breast sometimes deteriorates when they are fed by bottle teat, so parents may choose to avoid a bottle and look for alternative delivery methods. These include syringes, supplementary nursing systems, open cups and sippy cups.

A supplementary nursing system is basically a way of getting the milk from its container into the baby without a teat, and while the baby is feeding at the breast – so it includes a fine piece of tubing which is taped to mum's breast so that the tube goes into the baby's mouth with the nipple. When the baby suckles at the breast they are rewarded with milk from the container as well as from mum's breast.

If a newborn baby needs a little more milk than they are able to take at the breast, whether because they have a feeding issue or because their blood sugar has dipped, then open cups, almost like straight-sided clear egg cups, are often used to provide the additional milk (whether expressed breastmilk or supplements of formula) to very new babies, or babies in the neonatal unit who are quite weak or premature, and the babies are bundled up, almost upright, and actually lap the milk from the tilted cup, a little bit like a kitten. However, once the infant is strong enough they often wriggle about a bit as they are being fed, and can even knock the cup from the adult's hand, potentially wasting the breastmilk and causing distress for everyone – so for this reason we do not advocate cup-feeding milk to babies who are healthy and able to 'get involved' in the feeding in this way.

Open cup-feeding is not really recommended for older healthy term babies who are not yet old enough to feed themselves, and babies from newborn to around seven months old do not have the necessary control to operate a sippy cup alone. Older babies can sometimes learn to cup feed themselves using cups with handles.

There's also a nifty little thing called a soft cup feeder, which has a really soft clear shovel-shaped 'nib', which fills with milk and allows babies to drink more easily than from a sippy cup or in many cases even a bottle.

For reasons of dental and oral health and development, guidance states that we should have nothing other than milk or water in a bottle or spouted cup, because of where sugars will pool in the infant's mouth and how this can influence tooth decay. Of course babies under 12 months should not be having anything to drink apart from breastmilk or formula milk or water anyway.

For more information on bottles and teats and things you might need to know, see Chapter 9. Whatever you do, try to make informed choices about the type of feed you are giving and the way it is prepared, as well as the way in which it is offered to your child.

A note about homemade formula

Although the formulations the formula companies use are closely guarded industrial secrets, there are recipes for homemade formula available on the internet. These include ingredients such as raw (unpasteurised) cows' milk, gelatin and yeast flakes (there are 14 ingredients in total in the Weston A. Price Foundation homemade formula recipe), or beef/chicken broth, organic liver and coconut oil. There are also recipes for fortifying commercial infant milks with egg yolks and cod liver oil.

Some people believe that a homemade product is healthier and cheaper than commercial formulas, and it is certainly true that adults eating mixed diets generally benefit from homemade, unprocessed options, which may be where the desire to make homemade formula has come from – perhaps particularly in parts of the world such as the USA where the regulations around the ingredients in infant milks are so much less strict than in Europe. However, if we look more closely at the homemade versions, they are much higher in protein, iron and Vitamin A than breastmilk or commercially produced formula. As we have already seen, there are very strict rules governing what needs to be in infant milks, and what should not be – and the homemade recipes also contain a number of potentially troubling ingredients such as egg and raw cows' milk, which are not recommended to be given to infants because of the risks of infection, allergy and malnutrition.

Please be aware that homemade formula could harm the health and growth of a baby. Anyone wanting to make homemade baby formula for an infant would need to be aware of all the possible nutritional implications of each ingredient in the recipe. If you are considering it, please speak to a health visitor or GP and consider asking for a referral to a paediatric dietician to discuss your plans.

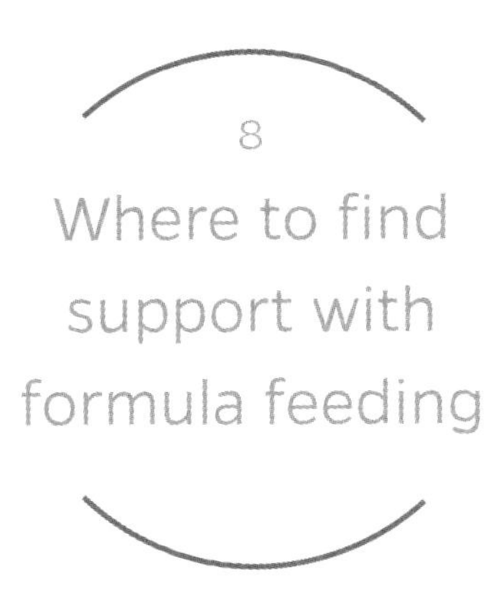

8 Where to find support with formula feeding

'I didn't think there was any formula feeding support – it was just the alternative to breastfeeding – and I frantically googled which formula and bottles to buy before we made a panicked trip to the supermarket. In hindsight I feel we really over fed R as a baby as we didn't know how to properly feed with a bottle.'
Amy, mum of two

While many parents feel there's little support available for formula feeding, actually health visitors will be experienced in dealing with simple formula feeding and bottle-feeding issues, although of course it's wise for any parent to inform themselves. One excellent source of impartial information is First Steps Nutrition Trust, which has really great evidence-based materials on its website www.firststepsnutrition.org about ingredients, types of milk and the evidence behind claims made for various specialist milks or ingredients.

Do be aware that the information on the websites of the formula manufacturers, or which are funded by formula manufacturers, is neither impartial nor robustly evidence-based. Clearly this goes for the information given by their phone lines too.

First Steps Nutrition Trust also has a guide to information provided online by those with funding from the sales of formula milks – find it by searching 'Websites and Organisations Funded by The Formula Industry'.

Sometimes health visitors and infant feeding co-ordinators have deliberately educated themselves in more depth about formula feeding and bottles (e.g. the different brands and types and their uses, and so on), and it's possible you will find someone able to work with you via your local NHS if you ask around. It is always worth making enquiries about free local support.

For more specialist support with particular feeding issues, or if there is no general support accessible locally, sometimes families pay to access paediatric dieticians or even IBCLCs (International Board Certified Lactation Consultants): this may seem odd, as the 'lactation' in the title might make you think that they only work with breastfeeding mothers, but actually this is the only qualification in common use in the UK that requires a firm understanding of the constituent ingredients of infant milks and what they might be intended to do, and a thorough understanding of how to resolve more complicated infant feeding issues, including bottle-feeding issues, reflux, colic, allergies and so on.

To find a local IBCLC – some are NHS, some voluntary and some in private practice – see the search facility on their professional organisation's website www.lcgb.org/find-an-ibclc. Check that anyone you have chosen to seek support from feels confident working on bottle/formula-feeding issues: some have more experience than others. All are expected to be non-judgemental and to work with the family to optimise the outcomes of whatever infant feeding process is chosen. Some IBCLCs, like me, can work remotely via video conferencing or social media platforms, and so can 'see' clients anywhere – it's worth looking around to see who is out there to help you. Of course the Covid-19 pandemic compelled everyone to look at online options more, so lots of us are very proficient now!

How to talk to healthcare professionals

Many health professionals involved in the world of new families pride themselves on their up-to-date knowledge and expertise in infant feeding, and will happily listen to, inform and support the families they work with to help them to achieve their goals. Unfortunately, the infant feeding world is also fraught with misunderstanding and misinformation, presented as fact. Sometimes we will want or need information from our health professional about how or what or when to feed our babies, and if we have heard scare stories from friends and family about what the midwife, health visitor, GP or IBCLC's opinions might be on the subject, we might be wary of raising our hands and asking that burning question.

The first thing we can do is make it clear that we are not looking for advice or opinion, but for *information and evidence* on which to base our choices. We can always ask for the evidence to support any recommendation that a healthcare professional may make.

If you can go into any encounter with some ideas yourself but with an open mind, and if you can do some research around the subject, so you are not completely reliant on the opinions offered by others, then you are likely to get the best outcomes.

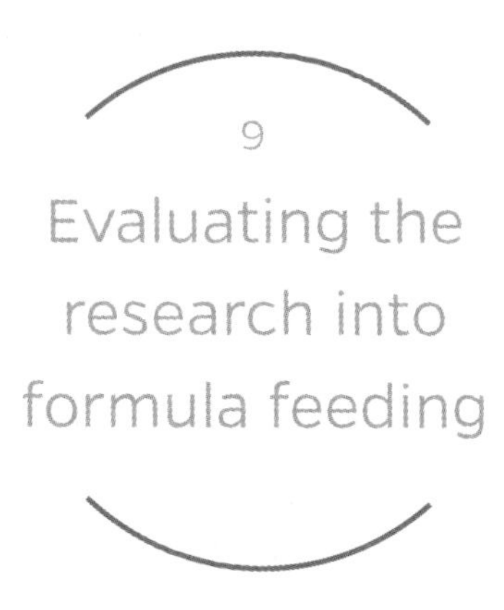

9
Evaluating the research into formula feeding

During your infant feeding journey, you may find that at times you want to look into a topic in more detail yourself, which might involve getting into the published research. There are a few things to be aware of when you begin to look at research into formula and formula-feeding.

Scientific research costs money, and tends to be financed by those who hope to see some financial benefit from it. For commercial products, like formula milk, research might uncover ways to make the product easier to sell, or more cost-effective to produce. Thus research on infant formula feeding is principally done by or paid for by the formula industry or the makers of specific ingredients. An exception is when paediatricians or others working with formula-fed babies have a specific hypothesis they wish to test – but often this research is still supported by the manufacturers of formula. None of the manufacturers hide the fact that the research into formula feeding is primarily conducted by them: indeed, all of the main players in the formula market in the UK proudly proclaim it on their websites and in their advertising.

'Aptamil is committed to exploring and understanding the wonderful and unique properties of breast milk. That's why our globally renowned scientists have been dedicated to pioneering research for 40 years.' Aptaclub website, July 2021

'..we have been researching the composition of breastmilk and its many components for over 50 years. We use this research, along with the work of many other experts and scientists from all around the world, to better understand what makes breastmilk so unique, and we use this information to help improve our milk formulas for babies when you cannot or choose not to breastfeed your baby.' Hipp Organic website, July 2021

'We have been leading research in baby nutrition for over 100 years and have produced a range of formulations expertly created with nature in mind to support babies' unique nutritional needs.' SMA Nutrition website, July 2021

The fact that most research is conducted by or financed by the formula companies means that parents and healthcare professionals who want to evaluate the scientific literature for themselves – either to inform their personal decision-making, or to help others find answers to questions they have – need to take into account the potential for bias and conflict of interest.

Most recent research into formula milk has focussed either on specialist products (so-called 'foods for special medical purposes' (FSMPs), such as the relatively expensive allergy or preterm formulas), or on what are known as 'novel ingredients', such as the new added nucleotides, oligosaccharides, probiotics and long-chain fatty acids. Before this there was some work done looking at protein levels in formula and the longer-term effects on growth rates (actually, it's been possible to analyse the protein levels in milk since 1883). This resulted in the protein levels in first infant milks being lowered, but it took a very long time to happen. And the reduction in protein levels has not been extended to many of the other products made by the same companies. The long-term effects of changes to formula milk composition are difficult to quantify, because it is unethical to carry out randomised controlled trials (RCTs) in infant feeding – it would mean *telling* a family whether they were to be in the 'exclusively breastfeeding' group, or the 'exclusively formula-feeding with standard formula' group, or the 'exclusively formula-feeding with new test formula', for example, which is obviously not on.

Consideration of nutritional adequacy

Current standards for infant formula focus on the safety of products, and on evidence for claims of benefit about specific ingredients. Ideally, the standards should require a demonstration of nutritional adequacy as well.

These standards for nutritional adequacy would then use indicators of the healthy development of infants – not the ingredients. As we know that there are risks to the infant from not breastfeeding, there is an argument that there has never been any infant formula which is nutritionally adequate. George Kent of the University of Hawai'i argues this in his work.

Furthermore, there are things in formula which are not in breastmilk – as Maureen Minchin writes:

> *'Industrially produced, dehydrated and multiply-heat treated powders always contain more than the original food they*

derive from. They also contain the products of processing, and traces of where those foods have hailed from, and how they were produced. We have got to get past seeing formula as a basically healthy food which just lacks some things, to seeing it as actually also containing many things of concern.

The harms of formula come not only from the absence of what's in breastmilk, but also from the presence of what's in formula, which Professor Paula Meier rightly said has 'separate detrimental effects': those pro-oxidants, chemical traces, contaminants, mould and bacterial spores, etc... Health professionals don't know enough about formula.' Maureen Minchin, December 2016

I don't say this to scare you, but because this knowledge is important for everyone involved in formula feeding, from the scientists to the consumers. Better knowledge will lead to better formula, as methods can be developed to reduce the ingredients of concern.

The problems of bias

When research is funded by baby food manufacturers, or other relevant non-independent sources, bias can creep in. This may be in the methods and conclusions of the research itself, or in the way in which the research is later used to support claims made in advertising. For example, sometimes the advertising of the product suggests health advantages which are not reported in the studies quoted, such as protection against gastrointestinal infections and allergy, which were not actually outcome measures in the studies used as references. First Steps Nutrition documents provide some good examples of this.

Claims for other benefits may be made without evidence to support them. For example, the claim made by a company rep my colleagues and I met with some years ago that 'thicker milk helps prevent babies from gulping in too much air' was not substantiated by the references provided, or by any evidence I have been able to find since. The use of thickened milks for infants with simple reflux is not supported by the ESPGHAN (European Society for Paediatric Gastroenterology, Hepatology and Nutrition) Committee on Nutrition, because there was no conclusive information on the potential effects of thickening agents on the bioavailability of nutrients and growth of children, or on mucosal, metabolic and endocrine responses (Aggett et al, 2002a).

Often studies on formula are small in scale, with very high dropout rates, very short follow-up periods and varying outcome measures. Sometimes they are large-scale but observational, with no randomisation and no control arm. Sometimes studies are well conducted and well reported, but the findings could be said to be only suggestive rather than conclusive, with only small effects and some problems with the design, for example only single-blinding (meaning that either the parents or the researchers in the trial knew which arm of the study they were participating in). Poor study design is common, and studies often refer to different milks of similar, but not the same, formulation.

Generalised findings

Sometimes research findings can only be generalised to high-risk infants, in whatever field the formula hopes to address – for example, those with family risk of allergy, or preterm babies. The findings should not be assumed to apply to the population as a whole, as they do not demonstrate effectiveness for babies who do not have the underlying condition specified in the research.

The opposite is also true: studies which show effects in the general population are used to provide evidence for products marketed for specialist needs. An example is a study by Kennedy et al, carried out in 1999. This was a well conducted and reported randomised double-blind study showing an increase in stool softness in infants fed the new formula. This should not be taken as 'decreasing constipation', as the participants were not constipated infants, and in fact the formula led to increased concern from mothers about runny poo.

Of course, formula companies have access to research on breastmilk too, either conducted by them, or by other groups. Studies have shown that lactic acid and bifidobacteria in breastmilk play important roles in the development of a healthy gut flora. Where the bias creeps in is when the companies use that work to suggest that strains of bifidobacteria in commercial preparations may be beneficial as supplements in infant formula, or make inferences about lactic acid in formula, when in fact that is not shown by the study.

Typically, research on formula compares one formula against another type of formula, or the same formula without the added ingredient, and does not include comparison with breastmilk or an analysis of babies who were mixed-fed breast and formula milk, even though there are often mixed-fed babies in the group. Remember that all formula advertising in the UK includes the opening statement 'breastfeeding is best for babies' and stresses the many years of breastmilk research. Why then does the research cited in support of these claims not include a comparison to breastmilk and breastfeeding? It is possible that they have omitted the analysis of infants who have been partially breastfed, where this may have had some protective effects, for example against atopic dermatitis or allergic rhinitis.

'Cherry picking' – the studies we don't see

It is a sad fact – for researchers – that despite huge investments of time, ingenuity and money studies often have disappointing or inconclusive outcomes. Arguably these are nonetheless useful studies, because they add to our wider understanding – but when that research is funded by a commercial company, often the results are shelved or suppressed. After all, why would a company publish a study showing a negative outcome for a product it makes? This situation makes it harder for organisations and independent academics to research formula and formula-feeding more fully, as they don't have access to a great deal of work that might be relevant.

Conflicts of interest in research

In recent years our understanding of the effects of conflict of interest in research has grown, and organisations like IBFAN (International Baby Foods Action Network) and the Conflict of Interest Coalition have been involved in highlighting where it exists. In infant feeding research there are always studies going on looking at new ingredients for formula milk, or new ways of formulating existing ingredients, involving many different researchers across the world. However, in the decade or more that I have been critically appraising the evidence base cited by formula companies to support their claims in advertising and marketing, I have seen the same names pop up quite a bit.

Examples include Prof Berthold Koletzko, who is a neonatologist in Munich in Germany, who has a special interest in the nutrition of preterm babies, and Prof Yvan Vandenplas, a paediatrician in Brussels in Belgium, who has a special interest in finding formula responses to cows' milk protein allergy. Both men have also been involved in producing company information and delivering study days and webinars for a formula manufacturer. A co-author on the Cochrane systematic review I was involved in writing on Dietary Modifications for Infantile Colic, published in autumn 2018, Dr Francesco Savino, a paediatrician in Italy who has been doing research into the effect of various strategies and formulations on reducing infantile distress and infantile colic, has authored many papers based on studies made with the assistance of formula manufacturers.

Another name which often pops up is that of Prof Michael Kramer from Canada, who is the lead author on the PROBIT study funded by the government of Belarus, which looked at the effectiveness of the implementation of Baby Friendly standards in hospitals there on improving breastfeeding rates and infant health outcomes. Over the years he has also worked on understanding febrile convulsions, the effects of various strategies for low-birth weight infants, nutritional advice for mothers in pregnancy to prevent allergy in at-risk children and exercise in pregnancy, among other topics. One large trial – led by another researcher with a large 'catalogue' of publications, Andrea von Berg, who is a researcher in paediatrics and immunology in Wesel in Germany – which includes Kramer among the co-authors, is described as:

> *'The German Infant Nutritional Intervention-Program (GINI) was supported for the first three years by the German Ministry for Education and Research… It is a birth cohort which was primarily scheduled until the children were 3 years old. The aim of the prospective, randomized, double-blind intervention study was to investigate the impact of different cow's milk protein hydrolysate infant formulas in the first 4–6 months on the development of allergic diseases in children at risk due to at least one parent or biological sibling with a history of allergic disease.'*

What is not clear from this outline is that the trial used formulas supplied by five different manufacturers. Nor does it say where the funding for the work came from after the first three years. However, the papers written have been used extensively by companies including Nestlé Nutrition to support changes made to the ingredients in some of their products in the UK.

What all this means for parents and healthcare professionals is that we need to be very careful when we evaluate evidence – not only looking at the study design, outcomes and reporting, but also at where the funding for the work has come from and who stands to benefit from the conclusions. Fortunately we are not on our own with this: many organisations and publications provide good summaries of the evidence, including First Steps Nutrition Trust, *The Lancet* Breastfeeding Series, the World Health Organization, and *Acta Paediatrica*.

What is the best sort of evidence?

In terms of the 'best' evidence, we all instinctively know that tests and trials and 'proper research' must be better than the opinion of your neighbour or someone you chat to in the supermarket, but in fact there is a *hierarchy of evidence*.

In 1997, Greenhalgh put the different types of primary study in the following order:

1. Systematic reviews and meta-analyses of RCTs with definitive results
2. RCTs with definitive results (confidence intervals that do not overlap the threshold clinically significant effect)
3. RCTs with non-definitive results (a point estimate that suggests a clinically significant effect but with confidence intervals overlapping the threshold for this effect)

4. Cohort studies
5. Case-control studies
6. Cross-sectional surveys
7. Case reports

Unless a case report, survey or particular individual study is used by industry to illustrate a point, or is particularly ground-breaking, it is unlikely to influence the practice of the majority of our healthcare providers – and this is not a bad thing, as single studies are not really robust evidence. The most robust types of evidence are the 'meta-analyses' or 'systematic reviews' – which analyse many different sources of information in a planned and methodical way.

Unfortunately, in formula marketing to health professionals the references used to back up claims may not be of high quality and may be very obscure. On one occasion colleagues and I tracked down a reference and discovered it was a poster presentation on a small study made at a conference, for which only a one-paragraph abstract exists! Numerous other references were to information that was 'on file' with the company, and not for general release.

This is at best misleading, and at worst an attempt to hide the reality of the research that has been done from healthcare professionals and the parents they work with.

Even well-conducted systematic reviews are only as good as the reviewers and the papers they are able to review – even the excellent templates, methodology and vigorous peer-review process of organisations like Cochrane cannot make a review immune to bias. The difference is that Cochrane insists on full conflict of interest (COI) declarations – although it does not stipulate that the authors must be *free* from financial conflicts of interest, just that they must *declare* them. For example, have a look at the first of three systematic reviews which I have co-authored about infantile colic (Gordon, M., Biagioli, E., Sorrenti, M., Lingua, C., Moja, L., Banks, S.S.C., Ceratto, S., Savino, F. 'Dietary modifications for infantile colic'. *Cochrane Database of Systematic Reviews* 2018, Issue 10). Googling the code CD011029 will take you there. At the end of the review you will find the declarations of interest – while I prefer to declare all rather than withhold, some of the other authors have chosen to declare no interests, one of them only refers to the three years prior to this publication and does not reveal previous connections, and another has interests with a particular manufacturer. I should stress that I am not saying that my co-authors on this review definitely did exhibit bias – I am simply using our own review as illustration of how disclosure works and how hard it can be to get the full picture.

What research do we need?

Consumers and health professionals would really benefit from up to date, brand-by-brand comparison studies of outcomes in formula-fed babies and older children, which continue into adulthood. These could measure simple things like weight gain, dental health, allergy and intolerance and measurable biological development, such as in brain and reproductive tissue.

In the longer term it would also be great to study the consequences of formula feeding for, for example, IQ and reproductive issues. These studies are simply not done, though there are good reasons why they should be – but clearly from an ethical perspective there are also reasons why we could not have the 'gold standard' randomised controlled trials.

All research on inflammatory disease in children or adults, in every organ, whether asthma, dermatitis, the brain or the gut, *could* routinely enquire about, document and report on the method of infant feeding of those with disease, and which brands and types of formula were used. But it doesn't. For things like obesity, irritable bowel disease, diabetes and autism we have some evidence that feeding method has an effect. But from a research point of view the questions are not being asked. This is an immense disservice to the families and children affected and future generations.

There should be regular independent monitoring in every country of heavy metals in formula milks, and of microbial presence in powdered formula as found in the tub, tin or carton, *and* as found in actual made-up mixtures which are being fed to our infants. I think most families expect that someone, somewhere, is keeping an eye on this stuff for us – and the sad reality is that they are not: it is left to industry to self-regulate.

Another useful and simple idea would be to document the formula supplementation of breastfed babies and the formula use of formula-fed-from-birth babies (amounts and brand) for every infant in every hospital in a permanent database. Many of the families I work with have no idea which formula their child was given in those early days, and there is certainly no centralised storage of this information to consult when there are problems. A similar system is required for donor breastmilk in the UK already (NICE Guideline CG93).

Finally, and it's hard to believe we do not already have this, all details of formula compositional changes, by brand and by date, should be recorded in a central permanent database. This would be helpful when unpicking what happens when formulation changes upset babies' guts – this happened with SMA in 2016 and Aptamil in 2018, and the reasons are still a mystery.

How does research evidence filter into practice?

When a new systematic review is published, it may attract media attention, or it may be added to the NICE Clinical Knowledge Summaries, but it takes time for even very robust and critically appraised meta-analysis of new evidence to make its way into frontline practice. It's an unfortunate fact that most health professionals in the UK are advising based on the evidence they were given when they trained, which may not have been completely up to date then. Only health professionals who take an interest in a particular area, spending their own money and time attending conferences, reading papers about research studies and trying to stay on top of news, are likely to be talking about the most up-to-date information we have. Unfortunately, some of the formula companies market their products direct to health professionals via 'free' study days at which they present evidence they have chosen.

Research about the risks of not breastfeeding

Health risks associated with the use of infant formula were first talked about in 1939 by Dr Cicely Williams, who warned against the dangers of using infant formula in low income countries without access to clean water and washing facilities, in a speech called 'Milk and Murder'. Since then, alongside the work on formula milk composition, scientists have been trying to investigate the health effects in mothers and babies who do not breastfeed.

As a provider of antenatal information about infant feeding in one of the areas of the UK with the lowest rates of breastfeeding, I often have to start conversations about pregnant women's thoughts about feeding their new baby. If the mother has never really thought about it, or has assumed that she would bottle-feed because that's all she has really seen, but is interested in knowing more so she can make her own decision, I usually try to find something that will resonate with her. This is because when I attended antenatal classes the first time I was pregnant, the mums-to-be researched the bonding and relationship-building aspects of feeding while the dads-to-be were sent off to research and report back on the health impact of feeding choices for both mum and baby. What was fascinating was how the chaps each chose to report back on something pertinent to their own family situation. For one it was about mum's risk of female cancers, as his mother had had ovarian cancer, while for another it was the risk of diabetes as the mum-to-be was suffering from gestational diabetes. For my own partner it was the risk of triggering eczema, which he had suffered with badly through his childhood and into adulthood. He wasn't interested in female cancers or diabetes as he didn't know anyone who had had them, but he was deeply invested in reducing his child's risk of the awful skin condition that he had suffered himself.

I realised then that there was no point trying a one-size-fits-all approach in providing antenatal information, because only certain arrows would hit their target. And no sense at all in talking about risks and benefits without all parties understanding what they mean.

To understand why *reduction in risk* doesn't mean something *won't happen to us*, we need to understand a bit more about risk and the factors that affect it.

> *'My mum breastfed three children and got breast cancer at age 53 unfortunately, so I've never really believed that it reduces your chance of getting breast cancer!'* mum-to-be on Babycentre

The most basic type of risk is *absolute risk*. Absolute risk is a person's chance of developing a certain disease over a certain period of time. It is estimated by looking at a large group of people who are similar in some way (the same age, for example) and then counting how many people in the group develop a certain disease over a certain period of time. Knowing the absolute risk of a disease can help us understand the health risks in our lives.

For example, the lifetime risk of developing breast cancer in 2020 was 1 in 7 for women in the UK, calculated by the Statistical Information Team at Cancer Research UK. This means that if we followed 1,000 women in the UK for their whole life, about 143 of them would develop breast cancer before death. According to Cancer UK (on their website, 2021), 8% of breast cancer cases in the UK are caused by overweight and obesity, 8% are caused by alcohol drinking and 5% are caused by not breastfeeding. Remember that breast cancer incidence is strongly related to age, with the highest incidence rates in older people. In the UK in 2018–20, on average each year a quarter (24%) of new cases were in people aged 75 and over. Age-specific incidence rates rise steadily from around age 30–34 and more steeply from around age 70–74. The highest rates are in the 85–89 age group. Many women of this age will not die *from* breast cancer, but may *have* breast cancer when they die.

Anything that increases or decreases a person's absolute risk of getting a disease is called a *risk factor*.

A risk factor can be related to things such as lifestyle (diet, smoking status, exercise), genetics (family history), reproduction (age at first period, pregnancies and breastfeeding history) and environment (exposure to toxins).

Some factors increase risk: older women have a higher risk of breast cancer than younger women, so age is a risk factor for breast cancer.

Some factors decrease risk: women who breastfeed have

a lower risk of breast cancer than women who don't, so not breastfeeding is also a risk factor for breast cancer.

However, because this is a *population-wide risk*, a slim, fit, non-smoking 40-year-old woman who breastfeeds all her five babies for a year each and has no family history of breast cancer can still get breast cancer, however small the risk may be, just as someone with a higher risk, for example a 90-year-old overweight woman who never breastfed and smokes a pack of cigarettes each day, may not get breast cancer. It is not about the *individual* but effectively about the *odds of the bet*.

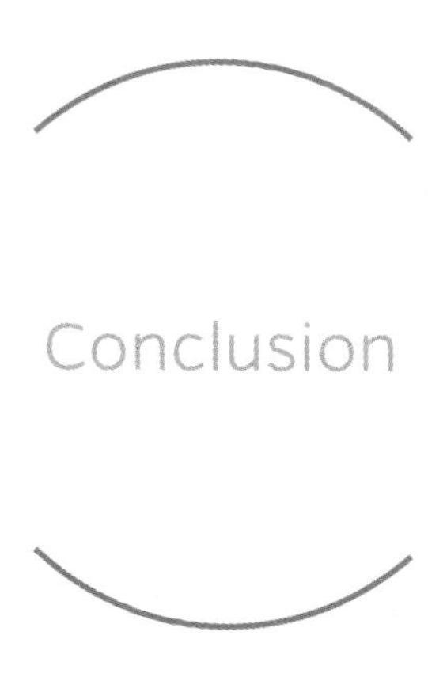

Conclusion

As this book draws to a close, I cannot put it better than Lisa, mum of four:

> *'What all parents want, regardless of how they feed their baby, is to be able to do the best job we can: we can only do that if we have the correct, evidence-based information with which to make truly informed decisions. The idea that new parents are delicate little flowers who cannot cope with the correct information is not only infantilising, insulting and patronising; but by obscuring the evidence-based information that we need in order to make truly informed decisions all society does is leave us at the mercy of the aggressive, predatory marketing "information" provided by companies who have a vested financial interest in persuading us we need their products.'*

I hope that this book has been able to answer a lot of the questions you had about formula, and perhaps has provided information – or even posed further questions – that you hadn't even considered.

One day, I hope that parents' choice of formula is facilitated by unbiased transparent sharing of information about the options available, and that formula milks are produced to the best standards possible and using the best quality products – which is the very least the youngest in our population deserve. Until that day, please continue to ask questions and please go into your decision-making with evidence-based information

Happy parenting!

Appendix:

A brief history of formula feeding

Late 1700s The industrial revolution saw more mothers in employment. A combination of wet nurses and 'pap' (bread, flour, sugar, water) was used for babies whose mothers were unable to stay at home and breastfeed them.

1835 Evaporated milk patented – before this there was no way to store and transport liquid milk.

1845 First rubber teat patented – before this, babies were fed via ceramic 'boats' or via glass bottles with cork or metal teats.

1860s First commercial infant formula 'Leibig's Perfect Infant Food' made in Germany (a liquid made from cows' milk, water, wheat flour, malt and potassium bicarb) and 'Leibig's Soluble Food for Babies' (a powder to be mixed with diluted cows' milk) launched, swiftly followed by a product from Henri Nestlé in Switzerland, which was a less expensive powder which could be mixed with water alone, and became the first internationally available powdered formula.

Early 1890s Scientists began to analyse the composition of breastmilk in an effort to make infant formulas more like human milk. The first changes included moving away from cows' milk fats towards a blend of animal and vegetable fats instead.

1919 The first, or at least most effective, of these 'humanised' milks with an added fat blend, was 'Synthetic Milk Adapted' – now known the world over as SMA.

1935 Reduction in protein level as ongoing study of breastmilk found that manufacturers had overestimated the levels of protein needed by the baby.

1941 National Dried Milk (withdrawn in 1976) introduced by the UK government: a dried, full fat modified cows' milk powder fortified with vitamin D.

1959 Iron-fortified powdered formulas introduced.

1962 Move from casein-based to whey-based formula, more like protein ratio of human milk.

1981 International Code of Marketing of Breastmilk Substitutes published by World Health Organization.

1984 Taurine first added to formula to help fat absorption – not yet required.

1988 Follow-on formulas first introduced to the UK market.

1990s Nucleotides added to enhance immune system development – not yet required.

1993 Long-chain polyunsaturated fatty acids introduced to aid growth – not yet required.

1995 Infant Formula and Follow-on Formula Regulations made law.

Late 1990s Probiotics (so-called 'friendly bacteria') added to some commercial infant formulas in Europe and across the world – now largely withdrawn in the UK.

2002 Government recommendations to use minimum 70°C water to make up formula from powder, owing to bacterial contamination.

2003 European Scientific Committee on Food (now known as EFSA) lists essential requirements of infant and follow-on formula.

2004 Prebiotics (FOS and GOS) first added, claimed to boost numbers of good gut bacteria.

2004 UK's Chief Medical Officer issues statement advising against use of infant soy formula.

2014 Goats' milk-based formula allowed in UK for the first time.

2014 European Food Safety Authority (EFSA) updates its infant and follow-on formula guidance to include minimum and maximum levels of ingredients.

2017 UK referendum on UK leaving the European Union – as at date of publication of this book, we still don't know how this may impact the marketing and safety guidance for infant milks.

2020 New regulations on composition, marketing and labelling set in 2016 came into force.

Further reading

www.researchgate.net/publication/313810831_Milk_Sharing_From_Private_Practice_to_Public_Pursuit

Why Breastfeeding Grief and Trauma Matter, Amy Brown, Pinter & Martin, 2019

Why Infant Reflux Matters, Carol Smyth, Pinter & Martin, 2021

Why Mothers' Medication Matters, Wendy Jones, Pinter & Martin, 2017

Milk Matters: infant feeding and immune disorder, Maureen Minchin

Let's talk about feeding your baby, Amy Brown, Pinter & Martin, 2021

Let's talk about your new family's sleep, Lyndsey Hookway, Pinter & Martin, 2021

The Big Letdown: How Medicine, Big Business, and Feminism Undermine Breastfeeding, Kimberly Seals Allers, St Martin's Press, 2017

The Politics of Breastfeeding, Gabrielle Palmer, Pinter & Martin, 2009

The Microbiome Effect: How your baby's birth affects their future health, Toni Harman and Alex Wakeford, Pinter & Martin, 2016

Why Tongue-tie Matters, Sarah Oakley, Pinter & Martin, 2021

Acknowledgements

To my kids, who've been raised by a mother dedicated to the pursuit of facilitating fully informed choice in others, which must make me a right pain to live with; and to all the friends I have made in the infant feeding world along the years, who have persuaded me that this book needed to be written – even if I didn't really have time.

Index

Available from Pinter & Martin
*in the **Why it Matters** series*

1. ***Why Your Baby's Sleep Matters*** Sarah Ockwell-Smith
2. ***Why Hypnobirthing Matters*** Katrina Berry
3. ***Why Doulas Matter*** Maddie McMahon
4. ***Why Postnatal Depression Matters*** Mia Scotland
5. ***Why Babywearing Matters*** Rosie Knowles
6. ***Why the Politics of Breastfeeding Matter*** Gabrielle Palmer
7. ***Why Breastfeeding Matters*** Charlotte Young
8. ***Why Starting Solids Matters*** Amy Brown
9. ***Why Human Rights in Childbirth Matter*** Rebecca Schiller
10. ***Why Mothers' Medication Matters*** Wendy Jones
11. ***Why Home Birth Matters*** Natalie Meddings
12. ***Why Caesarean Matters*** Clare Goggin
13. ***Why Mothering Matters*** Maddie McMahon
14. ***Why Induction Matters*** Rachel Reed
15. ***Why Birth Trauma Matters*** Emma Svanberg
16. ***Why Oxytocin Matters*** Kerstin Uvnäs Moberg
17. ***Why Breastfeeding Grief and Trauma Matter*** Amy Brown
18. ***Why Postnatal Recovery Matters*** Sophie Messager
19. ***Why Pregnancy and Postnatal Exercise Matter*** Rehana Jawadwala
20. ***Why Baby Loss Matters*** Kay King
21. ***Why Infant Reflux Matters*** Carol Smyth
22. ***Why Tongue-tie Matters*** Sarah Oakley
23. ***Why Formula Feeding Matters*** Shel Banks

Series editor: Susan Last

pinterandmartin.com